HOMOEOPATHY RECONSIDERED

A New Look at Hahnemann's Organon

BY THE SAME AUTHOR:

HOMOEOPATHY — A PATIENT'S GUIDE

HOMOEOPATHY RECONSIDERED

A New Look at Hahnemann's Organon

by

ANNE M. CLOVER
MBBS DPM FFHom.

LONDON
VICTOR GOLLANCZ LTD
1989

First Published in Great Britain 1989
by Victor Gollancz Ltd
14 Henrietta Street, London WC2E 8QJ

British Library Cataloguing in Publication Data
Clover, Anne M.
  Homoeopathy reconsidered.
  1. Medicine. Homeopathy
  I. Title   II. Hahnemann, Samuel, *1755–*
  Organon der Heilkunst
  615.5'32

  ISBN 0–575–04458–6

Typeset at The Spartan Press Ltd,
Lymington, Hants
and printed in Great Britain by
St Edmundsbury Press Ltd, Bury St Edmunds, Suffolk

This book is dedicated
to Eugene Halliday
in gratitude for his help
in its preparation

CONTENTS

BIBLIOGRAPHICAL NOTE

In the references at the end of each chapter, where no specific publication or translation is given, the material concerned appears in all published versions of the specified edition. Particular references are to the following books:

Haehl, Richard, *Samuel Hahnemann. His Life and Work*, Vol. I, The London Homoeopathic Publishing Company, 1922

Hahnemann, Samuel, *Chronic Diseases*, New Delhi, Jain Publishing Company

—— , *Organon of Medicine*, 6th Edition, trans. Dudgeon and Boericke, Calcutta, Roy Publishing House, 1970

—— , *Organon of Medicine*, 6th Edition, trans. Künzli, Naudé and Pendleton, Victor Gollancz Ltd, 1983

PREFACE

IN THE PRESENT decade, in which sophisticated surgery and complex pharmacy frequently become media headlines, it is hardly surprising that there is a widespread expectation that for most of our medical needs there should be an effective medical answer. It is a situation very different from that existing in the late seventeen and early eighteen hundreds when Samuel Hahnemann was doing the pioneer work that has played such an important role in the development of contemporary homoeopathy. In his time many diseases were accepted as incurable or, if considered treatable, likely to involve highly unpleasant procedures. The fashionable therapies of that era included purging, blood-letting and heavy doses of medicines such as arsenic and mercury. It was a far cry from the intricate surgery and precise pharmacy available now. Although unease is often voiced about the side-effects of many contemporary treatment regimes, or about the ethical issues they raise, most of us have cause to be grateful for the advances of modern medicine.

It may therefore be expected that the medical literature of the early eighteen hundreds is unlikely to be of much use today. What value, we may ask, can there be for us in the writings from the purging and blood-letting era? Obviously many such works are now reduced to historical interest. There are however exceptions which refer to principles as valid today as yesterday and to practices still widely found effective, safe and easily applied. Many people would say that amongst such works are the writings of Samuel Hahnemann, who was born in Saxony in 1755 and subsequently trained as a linguist, chemist and translator as well as a physician. Arguably, both his scientific work in developing the methods for preparing and prescribing homoeopathic medicines, and his philosophic enquiry into the related principles, are as valid today as they were over a century ago.

The purpose of this book is to look again at these principles, particularly as presented in the sixth and final edition of the *Organon of Medicine*, the major work by Hahnemann concerned with the principles of the nature of disease and its effective treatment by homoeopathy.

CHAPTER I

The Aims of Therapy

TWO QUESTIONS WERE recurrently considered by Samuel
Hahnemann throughout his long medical career. Born in
Saxony in 1755 he trained as a physician and subsequently
practised medicine in various European cities until his death
in Paris in 1843. Throughout his career he energetically
pursued two questions fundamental to all medical work. He
asked first, what is the nature of disease, and second, how
therefore can it be effectively and safely treated. His
continuing search for answers to these basic enquiries are
shown in his copious writings recording his detailed observations of patients and his interpretations of the data they
presented. Other training that aided Hahnemann's work
concerned subjects as diverse as linguistics and chemistry.
His extensive knowledge of languages facilitated his
widespread reading; his skill as a chemist proved useful in
his research and development of methods for producing safe
and effective medicines. His work incorporating these
abilities was to become the basis of modern homoeopathic
medicine.

Amongst the written records of Hahnemann's medical
practice are six editions of the *Organon*. These books are
particularly concerned with Hahnemann's searching questions concerning diseases and the therapies applied in hopes
of their correction. The six editions show his progressive
clarification of ideas concerning the nature of diseases and
their therapy.

Throughout all of his work Hahnemann argues the
importance of therapy being "rational". His first edition of
the *Organon* was called the *Organon of the Rational Art of
Healing*. Hahnemann's use of this term implies that the

practice to which it refers is well reasoned, has a rational basis before it is applied in practice. A contrary approach is often described as "empirical". That is, if something is found to be effective in practice it is used again with less emphasis on the details of why or how it works and more stress on the recall that it has previously appeared effective. Many times in his writings Hahnemann argues against such an empirical approach, and for the contrary method of first seeking to understand disease and then deducing an effective treatment for it. His third stage is to test his ideas in practice. This does not imply that he down-graded the value of practical experience. Quite the contrary, he frequently argues its importance. It is simply that he is saying, first clarify your principles, then apply them in practice. This book will examine his pursuit of this ideal and how it leads him to detailed questioning of how disease occurs, then to a study of medicines that can treat this process, and finally to a consideration of their application. It will refer mainly to Hahnemann's mature ideas as presented in his later works, particularly the sixth edition of the *Organon*.

Basic to all his questioning is Hahnemann's insistence on looking for the hidden causes of apparently obvious symptoms or physical changes. In his assessments of disease processes and their therapy he emphasizes that what we see with our ordinary eyes is merely the outer show, whilst less obvious but similarly important energies are operating behind the scenes to produce this effect. Today such an understanding is readily supported by science as well as by our own experience. We know in our own bodies that the unseen energies of emotion, thought or personal choice make a difference to our physical performance. If we are actively interested in a course of action, enjoying it and thinking clearly about its various aspects, the effect is very different from an apparently similar form of behaviour in which we are uninterested, irritated or bored. Such results of our inner motivation can be masked by training when we are adults; but in young children, so far relatively free from such restraint, their effects show particularly quickly. Such children often illustrate very clearly the effect interest or its lack can have on overt behaviour.

A contemporary scientific support for such awareness comes from physics. It has been clearly shown that our bodies and all gross structures, although they appear to be material entities, are in fact fields of energy or power behaving in a way that makes them look like a solid form. All substantial forms are composed by atoms which we now know to be energy phenomena. The collection of these in a human body, or a medicine able to treat it, is therefore a particular version of such dynamic activity. With this idea in mind it is much easier to understand that the energies we experience as thoughts and feelings are always interacting with the food and other forces we absorb from our environment to produce our physical form. Our bodies are like diverse currents converging in a unified stream.

Hahnemann was not the pioneer of such insights. Many other thinkers had referred to such an understanding long before the nineteenth century. Philosophers and religious thinkers from the earliest civilizations have referred in various ways to the continued interaction of the psyche and soma (or body) and argued therefore that both need consideration for a thorough assessment of disease and how to treat it.

How then does Hahnemann pursue and apply such ideas in homoeopathy? Throughout his writings he consistently argues that all symptoms of disease, though important, are only a visible front, or superficial aspect, of the hidden processes that give rise to them. That is, they are the outward signs giving evidence of the inner mechanisms. Consequently, he says, it is useless merely to try to ease these superficial effects. The greater need is to trace the inner cause and rectify this, so that the surface effects, or symptoms, are cleared at source.[1]

He is arguing, therefore, for attention to a basic polarization, or pairing, of apparent opposites. The seeming opposites here are the gross body and the hidden or causal forces that produce it. Always, he says, we need to attend to both aspects of this polarization, or pairing.[2] Throughout the six editions of the *Organon*, he strongly expresses his view of the inadequacy, as well as the danger, of looking at one aspect without the other. To try to assess the physical without due attention to the hidden forces that today we would term psychological and spiritual, is material bias.[3] On the other hand, he says that fanciful ideas not adequately applied to gross experience are mere empty speculation.[4] In colloquial language we could say you cannot have one without the other.

Hahnemann does not stop at saying simply that there are hidden roots as well as obvious and superficial symptoms of disease. In all his writings and particularly in the sixth edition of the *Organon*, he attempts to clarify an understanding of the various aspects of both of the poles of experience.

In relation to the more easily seen physical pole, he refers to the influence on disease of diet, exercise and housing, etc., noting their importance long before the need for public health was generally acknowledged. When he turns his attention to the hidden dynamics that interact with such physical dimensions he refers frequently to the vital force, a concept we will discuss shortly, and other influences that today we may describe as psychological or spiritual. It is as if all the time Hahnemann is saying watch for subtle factors and the hidden causes of disease, but at the same time do not forget the drains etc . . .[5] All of these aspects will be discussed in more detail later in this study. They are introduced here in the hope that an initial survey will facilitate a subsequent more detailed review.

When this polarized assessment of the causes of disease is applied therapeutically by Hahnemann he consistently refers to three stages. These too are summarized in the early paragraphs of the *Organon* and expanded later. He says that first we need to understand disease, what it is and what causes it. Secondly, we need to look closely for the powers hidden within medicines. Thirdly, we can then deduce how to apply the medicinal powers for effective treatment of disease processes. In other words, he is saying, first discover the details of a disease process; second, carefully investigate the medicines that can correct it and then, third stage, put the first two together for safe, effective treatment. This threefold approach, introduced at the beginning of the *Organon*, sets the plan for its contents. In the sixth edition paragraphs 1–71 are a review of the principles basic to homoeopathy and this threefold approach. The following paragraphs, that is 72–294, are clearly designated to the three stages. 72–104 consider a knowledge of disease; 105–145 a knowledge of medicines; and 146–294 their application. In each of these stages Hahnemann pursues an understanding of the polar aspects of gross and causal to which he refers in the opening paragraphs of the *Organon*.

Such an outline of the *Organon* will, I hope, serve as a background guide as we now begin to look in more detail at Hahnemann's understanding of homoeopathy, particularly as presented in the *Organon*.

Hahnemann begins by stating his view of the aim for a physician. In his characteristically dogmatic style he states that the only aim for a physician is to restore health. Perhaps it was an intended challenge to some of his more conventional medical colleagues who on many occasions he accused of damaging or even ruining the health of patients.[6] After stating this therapeutic aim in the opening paragraph of the *Organon* he immediately expands it by requiring in the next paragraph that the return to health should be quick, gentle, as harmless as possible, long-lasting and based on understandable principles. He then introduces his threefold approach to the pursuit of this ideal. We will see how Hahnemann's progressive discussions of these aims lead him to the conclusion that they are most likely to be achieved through homoeopathy.

Early in his research and practice Hahnemann started using the term homoeopathy to refer to the principle basic to the therapeutic method he claimed to discover. It was made up from two Greek roots, *homoios*, implying like or similar, and *pathos*, suffering. Together, therefore, the two root forms implied the use of agents that can produce in a relatively healthy person symptoms similar to those it can treat in one who is sick. It is often paraphrased today as being a system of using likes to treat likes. Or, in colloquial terms, "having a hair of the dog that bit you". This principle of similars, as it is sometimes described, remains the basis of homoeopathic practice. It will be referred to recurrently throughout this study as well as being the main subject of the sixth chapter.

Hahnemann deduced the similia principle after a personal experiment performed in about 1790 intended to demonstrate the medicinal effects of cinchona bark.[7] He found that it produced in him symptoms similar to the effect of malaria even though he had not previously had this disease himself. He also knew from his medical training that it could treat malaria. Putting these two together he deduced the principle fundamental to his subsequent practice. He then went on to research and test it out on himself, his friends and family, and later applied it for patients.

Through all such work, Hahnemann pursued his intent to observe the subtle and hidden, as well as the gross and obvious effects, both of diseases and the medicines applied in their therapy. We shall see how he argues that the rightly selected homoeopathic remedy, termed by him the simillimum, could provide the right stimulus to rectify hidden causes of disease and thereby assist the required healing.

First, however, we will look in more detail at the implications of Hahnemann's stated aim for a therapeutic process, namely the quick, gentle and lasting restoration of health, and how this relates to his consistent emphasis on the polarized aspects of the human body. This is of such fundamental importance to Hahnemann's work that it warrants careful attention here right at the beginning of this review. Hahnemann states many times that the physical state of health or disease is merely a front to hidden, unseen processes. We could liken it today to the skin of a child's balloon that implies the pressure of air inside it to maintain its shape. In referring to these hidden energies Hahnemann frequently uses a term widely employed in his day but probably unfamiliar to many people now. That is, the "vital force". In Hahnemann's time this phrase implied the energies believed to enliven the human organism, hence the term "vital". It described the power experienced as compelling the living activity of an otherwise apparently inert material form.

Unfortunately to Western ears such terms are often interpreted in a dualistic, or two-way, manner, with the opposing aspects seen as separates. This apparent separation is heightened when, as commonly happens today, more attention is paid to the physical body state and less to the hidden energies that support it. Such an emphasis remains apparent in many branches of medical practice today. It also shows itself in such common phrases as "it does not matter what you think, just get on and do it". Probably most parents have said this in exasperated moments at some stage, but if we look carefully at its implications we will see that it again indicates the idea that unseen mental activity can be separated from obvious physical performance. Technological medicine falls into a similar trap when disease is assessed and treatment devised with appropriately careful attention to physical processes, but insufficient respect to their concurrent psychological aspects. Science, as well as our own experience, reminds us today that unseen thoughts and feelings, as well as obvious physical influences such as food and exercise, all the time contribute to how we perform. Hahnemann said it long ago when he discussed the role of the unseen vital force in determining physical symptoms or health. Today we are more likely to refer to such a hidden driving force by talking of subconscious psychological energies or processes.

His discussions of these hidden causes of disease probe even further when he looks at the role of "spiritual" or "conceptual essences".[8] Hahnemann wrote in German, and

the words "Geistartigen Wesen", since translated conceptual or spiritual essence, appear particularly in the later
editions of the *Organon*. They are not easily understood but
appear to imply an insight concerning initiatory forces, that
is, the beginnings or prime movers of the heirarchy of
energies that we see operating in our bodies and in their
environment. The term spirit is used in many different ways
today but its roots imply an original intention, the beginning
of a process. Some of the religious interpretations have
unfortunately at times been presented in a dogmatic manner
that has hindered careful search for precise implications.
Philosophers and other thinkers have also often used the
term, here attempting to imply the initiative or primary
vector of a particular course of action.

So far, then, we are observing an hierarchy or spectrum of
causes discussed by Hahnemann in his determination to
understand disease. Whilst he stresses the importance of
checking for physical symptoms and their similarly gross
causal factors, such as inappropriate diet, drainage or drugs,
he is also looking at the effects of the vital force or hidden
psychological determinants and, on an even more subtle
level, trying to understand the original intention or choice
that sets the process in motion. He is therefore examining the
physical effects and at the same time trying to understand
the psychological and initiatory processes that influence
them. It is a wide-ranging as well as detailed review,
constantly seeking to understand the polar aspects of hidden
causes of visible effects.

This polarized assessment is fundamental to all his further
discussions, particularly in the *Organon*, of details concerning
the nature of diseases, medicines that can treat them and
their judicious employment. All the time he is expanding the
initial aim he has set for himself, namely to heal the sick,
while constantly repeating that for this to happen there has
to be due acknowledgement of all the relevant factors.
Hahnemann's concept of cure is concerned with far more
than merely removing symptoms. He states many times that

a thorough cure requires assessment of all the causal factors involved and their rectification. Only then, he argues, can symptom removal be complete. Anything less than this he describes as suppression and cover-up.

He terms such a cure a restoration to health.[9] His use of these terms to qualify his view of therapy has interesting implications. They suggest that Hahnemann regarded successful therapy as returning an individual to an ordered or balanced function, an original condition impaired in disease. The words health and healing come from Greek roots denoting wholeness. The restoration sought by Hahnemann therefore refers to returning to an appropriate interfunction of all the aspects of the person. He regards healthy function as a state to be rediscovered and only accepts it as attained when he sees correct physical function balanced with due sensitivity, clear assessment and responsible individual choice.

In other words, he is arguing that the ultimate aim of therapy is for human beings to reorganize their hidden potential, or, as the Delphic Oracle says, "Know thyself" and, as Shakespeare says, "Become what thou art". This is Hahnemann's stated aim for therapy.[10] Of course he seeks removal of unpleasant or inconvenient symptoms. But at the same time he is arguing the need to understand them in order to treat them thoroughly, and reminding us that such insight not only eases sickness but can help man recognize the deeper realities of his own being. It is a high aim.

The following chapters will trace Hahnemann's pursuit of this ideal together with his research into the homoeopathic process.

REFERENCES

1. *Organon* 6th Edition   Paras 7, 15–17
2. Ibid.   Paras 7, 7a, 7b
3. *Organon of Medicine.*   Introduction pp. 48–51 trans. Dudgeon and Boericke

4. *Organon* 2nd Edition   Preface

5. *Organon* 6th Edition   Paras 73–77

6. *Organon of Medicine.*   Introduction trans. Dudgeon and Boericke

7. *Samuel Hahnemann. His Life and Work.*   Haehl Ch. 5

8. *Organon* 6th Edition   Paras 20, 269 and footnotes, 270 and footnotes

9. Ibid.   Paras 2, 12, 17

10. Ibid.   Para. 141a

CHAPTER II

The Nature of Disease

WITH THE USUAL emphasis in the West on material aspects of experience it is not surprising that disease is often seen in predominantly physical terms. With infections the emphasis is on small organisms and their effects, with accidents it is on gross trauma and how it affects the victim, and with "degenerative", or wear and tear diseases, it is on how the physical changes limit physical function. Even with psychological problems, such as anxiety or depressive illnesses, there is growing attention to chemical changes in the body and how they appear to be associated with the symptoms presented. Whilst due care obviously has to be paid to such factors it is not helpful if they assume such prominence that other determinants are obscured.

Such opinions are not denying the value of the intricate assessments of disease effects often made in medicine today. Obviously increased learning about anything rightly used can only be helpful. The unease felt by many people today about the material aspect of much of Western medicine is because of the emphasis placed on the obvious effects of disease. Many people feel that whilst the learning itself can be highly beneficial, it can also become a hindrance if it detracts from other aspects of the process that also need attention. For instance, someone with an acutely inflamed appendix will usually be very grateful if it is efficiently removed. But, if at the same time their individual reactions to it, their anxiety about an operation, their concern for family needs, as well as their personal psychological conflicts that may have contributed to their illness, are ignored, they may well also react with a sense of frustration.

As we have seen, Hahnemann's view of disease strongly

opposes such a materialistic bias and constantly argues the need for a comprehensive review of its processes. Whether disease is presented as an apparently superficial skin rash, or as a deeply invasive cancer, to him the symptoms implied far more than the physical effects as reported by patients, their relatives or physicians. It is an emphasis that usefully counters the materialistic bias, or blinkers, often evident in many forms of contemporary medicine.

Fundamental to all such detailed assessments of disease by Hahnemann is his awareness of the primary polarization, that is, the pairing of easily seen physical effects and unseen psychological or spiritual causes. We have already referred to this interaction and will pursue it further now.

Like many theorists before and after him, Hahnemann argues that, just as the cosmic order is maintained by unseen geophysical forces, similarly the human order is maintained by unseen directives, such as the vital force and spiritual essences. From the earliest paragraphs of the *Organon* Hahnemann applies such concepts in assessments of human disease and at the same time introduces a note of caution. While he specifies hidden factors such as emotions, ideological conflicts and family pressures that may contribute to disease, he also warns against ill-founded speculation on their role.[1] That is, he strongly opposes consideration of subtle causes of disease without due reference to the symptoms that he regards as their product. After introducing this note of caution he summarizes his assessment by saying, "It is the totality of symptoms, *the outer image expressing the inner essence of the disease, i.e. of the disturbed vital force*, that must be the main, even the only, means by which the disease allows us to find the necessary remedy."[2] This statement and others like it clearly show Hahnemann's two-way appraisal of the nature of disease, with due attention both to the physical symptoms and the hidden factors producing them. It is like trying to understand the gross exterior structure of a steam engine together with its hidden power source.

Disease, Hahnemann argues, is always due to an "untunement", as he terms it, of the vital force.[3] The same vital force, he reminds us, is just what the term implies, vital or life-giving. It maintains the health of the whole body. But these forces, when disordered for any reason, become the source of disease. He therefore describes disease as a "dynamic untunement", and symptoms, whatever their form, as its peripheral effects.[4] It is like seeing a tree with new leaves unfolding, and remembering the unseen forces that support it. This description of inner and outer aspects of a disease process is merely the beginning of Hahnemann's classification. From this starting-point he delves progressively deeper, clarifying particular aspects of both poles of this spectrum.

In relation to outer changes he assesses the particular symptoms in minute detail, noting their type, order of development, time pattern after they are established, together with a meticulous assessment of their position in the body, their quality and effect on function. Details of patients' reports were then combined with his own examination.

His assessment of the inner or unseen aspects was similarly careful and detailed. Hahnemann openly states his understanding that disturbing emotional imprints, restrictive ideas and other memories held by a person can play a major role in the development of physical symptoms.[5] He appears to regard these as aspects of the vital force or dynamis, the hidden influence which he frequently says provokes visible symptoms. Today we could describe them as unseen psychological causes of recordable physical effects.

At the beginning of this century the widely publicized work of Sigmund Freud drew attention to the influence that recorded feelings and ideas can exert on the subsequent behaviour of human beings. Since Freud, it has become progressively more fashionable to try to understand the part they play in producing disease and to find ways consciously to change them. Of course, there is still opposition to such insight from people who prefer not to acknowledge the relevance of psychological vectors, or disagree with Freud's assessment of their role. But, overall, there is more understanding of the importance of such inner dynamics. The terminology has progressed since Freud, with more use today of reference to imprinting. But whether we use Freudian-type terminology and speak of subconscious and repressed data, or talk of subrational energy imprints, either way we are implying recorded ideas, feelings and other memory traces that are retained from past experiences but assert their effect now. It is as if the human body is a large, specially designed tape-recorder able to replay today the recordings of previous times, representing not only the forms of these but also the emotional changes associated with them.

Obviously, this can have a useful function. An imprint can remind us to look left-right-left before crossing the road, or how to work the controls if we are in a car using that road. This is clearly a useful and economical training measure. But like most experiences this recording capacity of the body can be harmful as well as helpful to us. Imprints can be restrictive or, as Hahnemann argues, can even become factors in the cause of disease. An example of this occurred in a young woman whose natural artistic ability was ignored after she abandoned painting following ridicule by her father. She became increasingly depressed. Her therapy included getting back to painting again as she gradually overcame the negative ideas that had previously restrained her. Hahnemann's illustrations include repression of natural sexual drive by over-vigorous moral training.[6] A rigid and repressive training, an over-emphasized inner "thou shalt not", can easily become a factor in the development of psychological or physical symptoms. Although Hahnemann did not use terminology familiar to most of us today, his writings clearly imply a similar understanding. Such influences, he argues, contribute to the unseen dynamism giving rise to the façade or front of visible symptoms.

Other inner determinants of symptoms discussed by Hahnemann include spiritual or initiatory forces. He often refers to hidden spiritual factors that influence all our physical activities. As a particular example he refers to the movement of an arm, reminding us that this occurs not only because of visible structures, such as bones and muscles, but because of the hidden intention causing their action.[7] These are searching ideas concerning fundamental causes of human behaviour in health or disease. They are not easy to understand but are clearly important if we are to pursue a thorough understanding of the determinants of human function. Hahnemann introduces them in the early paragraphs of the *Organon* and subsequently refers to them in progressive detail. This study will follow a similar pattern and further discuss such insights in later chapters.

So far we have observed Hahnemann's persistent concern with the two polar aspects, the seen and the unseen, of our health or disease. In addition we have noted some of his references to various modalities of the unseen psychological vectors. Observation of an implicit five-fold hierarchy helps to clarify this assessment. Its highest level is the inner spirit or individual capacity for choice illustrated by Hahnemann's reference to the act of will involved in moving an arm.[8] Next there are the energies of reason, a capacity to reflect on and understand our behaviour.[9] A third aspect consists of more particular thought processes about the specific experience of the moment and whether or not this integrates with the prior understanding and aim we have developed.[10] A simple example today would be calculating whether or not a chocolate offered for eating now would support or oppose an understanding of a need to diet. Fourth, there are emotions which may welcome or oppose the present activity because of remembered likes and dislikes.[11] Using the chocolate example again, a person may recall liking the taste, but disliking an after-effect, such as migraine if they react this way. All of these modes of function, Hahnemann argues,

27

contribute to the physical state of relative health or disease, which is the fifth level.

Such theories probably sound less strange to our ears today than was likely in Hahnemann's time. Today the media frequently produce dramas, documentaries or news reports referring to the physical effects of psychological trauma. As we noted earlier, this is part of our post-Freudian culture. Hahnemann was about 100 years pre-Freud. It shows his ability to be forward-thinking.

Another stage in Hahnemann's developing insight is shown when he pursues the idea that these disease processes are a lapse from an ideal order originally present in a human being. We noticed this briefly in chapter I in referring to the implications of Hahnemann's stated aim for a physician, namely the restoration of health. It appears that he saw disease as a deviation from a prior order, with the vital force and spiritual aspects of the individual person in some way altered from their own ideal state to produce conflict and disease. For a return to health there is therefore a need for restoration of this inherent order. That is, a restoration of balance between the initiative (or spiritual aspect), the vital force, and the physical energies. Such a restoration, Hahnemann argues, can be provoked by a correctly applied homoeopathic stimulus. That is, one selected according to the principle of similars, fine enough to interact with the subtle causes of disease and strong enough to provoke their correction.[12]

In such discussions concerning the nature of disease Hahnemann always emphasizes the individuality of the process.[13] While the principles have a general application for everyone, they are unique in their presentation by a person at any moment.

This theme always accompanies Hahnemann's polarized assessment of disease and he applies it consistently in his writings and practice. It is shown particularly clearly when he gives detailed instructions on how to assess the individual needs of patients seeking homoeopathic help. To illustrate his directions he refers to the hazard of using particular names for diseases and reminds us, for instance, not just to take note of "St Vitus Dance", but "a *kind* of St Vitus Dance".[14] Applying this insistence on individual assessments of diseases more familiar today, we would say that we need to look for individual features of "tonsillitis" or "hay fever" and not merely assume we know precisely what is happening in someone by saying they have such named conditions. Any disease, no matter how common, is individual to the patient at that moment in time. Consequently, a review of a person's symptoms, pursued in the manner advised by Hahnemann, will always note their individual features as well as patterns perhaps shown by many others with apparently similar complaints.

Such a requirement is a challenging ideal and was probably a major cause of the long queue of carriages said to have lined up in Paris when people were waiting to consult Dr Hahnemann. But clearly it is essential to a thorough assessment of disease and subsequent search for an individual remedy. It is an emphasis by no means unique to homoeopathy. Many branches of contemporary medicine also aim for such an individual assessment. Unfortunately many others also obscure it.

It is not surprising that Hahnemann's strong emphasis on prescribing according to individual needs has appealed to many patients. We know intuitively our own uniqueness. Evolution has outgrown the herd mentality and tribal era and instead we are now in the age of individuality. It is a basic factor that has probably been a major cause of the growth of interest in homoeopathy in recent years.

In Hahnemann's assessment of the nature of diseases we therefore find these two themes developed concurrently. That is, that the observed effects of diseases always imply hidden causes, and secondly, that the presentation of the process is always unique to the individual patient. Both in the preliminary and subsequent chapters of the *Organon* these themes are discussed in progressive detail. The early references to the polarized and individual nature of all diseases are like the superficial layers of the therapeutic onion. The next chapter will attempt to peel back further in tracing Hahnemann's progressive insights into the details of how and why disease occurs.

REFERENCES

1. *Organon* 6th Edition   Paras 5–7
2. *Organon* 6th Edition   Para. 7 trans. Künzli, Naudé and Pendleton
3. Ibid.   Paras 11, 22a, 29, 31a
4. *Organon* 6th Edition   Paras 7–15
5. Ibid.   Paras 77, 81a, 93a, 224, 225
6. Ibid.   Para. 81a
7. Ibid.   Para. 11a, final sentences
8. Ibid.   Paras 9, 11a
9. Ibid.   Paras 9, 61, 62
10. Ibid.   Paras 17a, 224a
11. Ibid.   Para. 225
12. Ibid.   Paras 16, 22, 26–28, 34
13. Ibid.   Paras 18, 82, 83
14. Ibid.   Para. 81b

CHAPTER III

The Causes of Disease

IN THE PREVIOUS chapter we compared Hahnemann's concern to understand the nature of disease to considering the power that drives a steam engine rather than merely using the thrust it affords. The analogy can be further pursued. If a steam engine fails, the cause has to be traced and corrected for its function to be restored. Disease, Hahnemann argues, is similar. The cause of the problem needs to be traced and corrected to achieve a thorough cure. In developing this assessment Hahnemann progressively reviews an hierarchy in the causal factors that he regarded as important.

When disease occurs many people try either to ignore it totally, or to ease its superficial effects in hopes of avoiding looking closer for its causes. Common examples of this are inappropriately using make-up to hide skin problems, or taking analgesics (pain-relieving tablets) to suppress unexplained symptoms. Hahnemann argues recurrently that to try and gloss over or ignore disease itself feeds the process. He observed that when patients tried either to forget symptoms and their causes, or merely sought to ease the superficial effects, the problems not only persisted, but often worsened. In his opinion one of the commonest factors causing diseases and complicating them was the attempt to ignore them. He therefore set out instead to trace their causes.

In his review of the causal factors involved, Hahnemann looks again at an hierarchy with drains and diets at its more obvious end, initiatory forces for its most subtle causes and other psychological or unseen environmental factors between the two extremes.[1] One way of clarifying this range of causal factors is to apply the five-level assessment of human function introduced in the previous chapter.

The natural tendency when assessing causes of disease is to look first for physical factors such as infectious organisms, and for environmental influences such as housing or climatic problems. The role of micro-organisms such as bacteria or viruses in causing diseases was hinted at by Hahnemann even though in his day they had not been discovered. He pays particular attention to such infectious agents when he discusses the causes of epidemic disease such as measles and smallpox and arguably anticipates the discovery to be made later of the precise organisms involved.[2] His views on the part such agents can play in the development of diseases are clearly important. They are relevant to his discussions both of acute epidemic diseases and also of the longer-lasting or chronic problems that he associated with lingering effects of certain forms of infection. We will look at them again in the next chapter.

It is evident from his many writings that Hahnemann recognized the importance of personal hygiene, suitable housing and appropriate regimes of diet, exercise and sleep, long before any other medical thinkers. With the emphasis placed on such concerns today, it may be difficult for us to imagine the lesser attention generally given to them in Hahnemann's era. Even in this respect he showed a pioneer mind and function when he emphasized their importance as possible contributory factors in the development of disease. He referred frequently, in his typically forthright manner, to the problems presented by inadequate ventilation or dampness of houses, deficient sleep or exercise and inappropriate diets. Sometimes Hahnemann's list of dietary ingredients that he said could contribute to disease was so long that you might wonder what remained on his menu. In general, he appears to have regarded too much of anything, particularly alcohol, coffee and tea, as well as deprivation or too little of the required food, as likely to induce disease. On the positive side, he advises simple food, not too stimulating, free if possible from what he calls medicinal herbs, and all this to be as fresh as possible.[3]

Closely related to these thoughts are Hahnemann's views on the misuse of drugs as a cause of disease. He saw the use of drugs in too high or too protracted doses as one of the common and avoidable factors. As particular examples he refers to the abuse of mercurial products, medicinal plant extracts such as the foxglove, and other groups of drugs such as stimulants, purgatives or sedatives.[4] His comments are still valid today when it is often observed that the abuse of various drugs can itself contribute to disease. Today, we are familiar with the addiction problems that arise with some of the tranquillizers such as Valium, or with stomach diseases that can be induced by taking too many aspirins, noting merely two of the common modern examples of this problem. As Hahnemann observed, medicines that in appropriate doses can be helpful, if taken in excessive amounts, can also be harmful. This again is generally better and more widely known today than was likely in Hahnemann's time.

The second level in the five-fold review of a causal hierarchy is concerned with emotions. When Hahnemann looks at these and their capacity to provoke disease he refers particularly to persisting negative or violent emotions as well as the effects of stress, anxiety and other disruptive emotional pressures.[5] I briefly noted in an earlier chapter that one way of illustrating this is to compare the human body to a tape-recorder. Just as the tape can record sound impressions, the cells of our bodies can hold memories of emotional pressures. This is far easier to understand now that science has shown us that all matter, including our physical body, is made of energy or patterns of power than can be moved by such emotional pressures. An interesting point worth noting here is that the word emotion itself implies movement (i.e. out-motion), reminding us that such forces are one flux reacting with the other patterns of energy in our bodies. The process is comparable to water colours mixing in a child's paint pot.

As well as deducing the role of emotional pressures in diseases, Hahnemann also went a stage further and discussed how such understanding could be applied therapeutically. This is emphasized particularly in his paragraphs on the treatment of mental illness in the latter sections of the *Organon* and again will be further discussed. But let us note at this stage that Hahnemann many times refers to the part emotional conflicts, retained in a person, can play in the development of any illness, that is, those with physical as well as mental symptoms. It is an important insight.

Closely related to emotions are thoughts, the third aspect in our five-fold review. The intellectual function has a defining role, it is an analysis and statement of sensations. Thoughts clarify what may otherwise be confused sensory impressions, whilst the quality of sensation enlivens what may otherwise appear to be a rigid analysis. It is a polarization evidenced particularly clearly in the sexual roles when men tend to stress definition and reason, and women the perception of subtle feelings. A common example occurs when men challenge women to think more carefully, while women are perceiving subtle feelings unnoticed by their partners. The two functions are complementary, with thoughts assessing and organizing the subtle feelings associated with physical activity. A healthy balance operates when we think clearly, feel sensitively and act decisively, with each of these three like equal sides of a triangle balancing one another. But, as we all know, such integration is not always maintained and unconscious over-emphasis can be given to any aspect of the triad.

When Hahnemann considers non-integrated thoughts and how they can cause disease he refers particularly to the effects of rigid moral training and the personal reaction to it.[6] The imprinting theory reminds us that our bodies hold impressions, or memory traces of past experiences. Among these are the ideas we learn as we grow up. They may be the result of quiet but frequent repetition, or forceful dictates, especially those backed up by threat of disapproval or punishment. One is like the slow steady water drip that gradually erodes resistant rock, the other like a disruptive waterfall. Either way a message is built into a body for certain standards to be attained.

Clearly an appropriate degree of such training is very important to our development. As is often said, everyone requires standards. Without them our ego structure, that is our personal sense of identity, would be unclear and lack direction. Obviously they have a fundamental and necessary role. But they can also be over-stated in a way that can be restrictive and a cause of conflict within our own person. An example is a child growing up in a home that discourages any sport. If, in later years, that child pursues an inclination to try a particular sport, it will conflict with the imprints from his earlier years and set up a battle in his own psyche. Another example can occur when teenagers from a home with a strong political bias oppose it and join up with another party. Again a conflict is likely within their own person. At times such reactions can be strong enough to cause obvious signs of disease. The body energies are sufficiently disturbed to produce easily seen symptoms that may have a physical or psychological emphasis, and perhaps require treatment.

As Hahnemann and many other researchers have said, if such tensions can be understood there is more chance of resolving them. It is possible to recognize and understand the conflict between past training and present initiatives, to express consciously at least some of the tensions provoked and then personally and deliberately choose which course to follow. When that happens one proves to oneself one's own inherent capacity to order one's own person.

Arguably Hahnemann was referring to such a possibility when he wrote of the "reason-gifted mind", as Dudgeon translates part of the ninth paragraph of the fifth and sixth editions of the *Organon*. The phrase implies an aspect of individual consciousness able to integrate the thoughts, emotional imprints and related data remembered from

35

previous experiences. When that happens the individual has organized his own energies and rebalanced at least some aspects of previously conflicting data.

Such discussions imply the fourth and fifth aspects of our five-fold assessment of human consciousness and the role of each of these in health or disease. The fourth is an overall understanding of how individual thoughts, emotional reactions and physical activities fit together. It is like seeing a view from the top of a hill and understanding a pattern of interaction between fields, roads, houses and people passed on the way up it. Such understanding then facilitates an informed choice of what action to take now. Instead of reliance on fragmentary data, there is an overall awareness that opens the way for an informed initiative. Such an initiative is the fifth level in the hierarchy. It is an ability to make a decision not biased by an assessment of the present situation that is only partial, or by particular aspects of past training taken out of context from other criteria. This does not imply that such an initiative will never co-operate with past training. Such apparent compliance may appear to occur when a person chooses consciously for himself to follow his prior training. But in this situation the choice is intentional and not a mere unquestioned repetition of old habits. An obvious example is still choosing to look left-right-left before crossing a road. We can choose to do this because we understand its advantages.

In many of his writings Hahnemann refers to the capacity for a human being to make his own informed choice. Such a choice of a course of action is an initiation, a beginning. A phrase in Hahnemann's later writings that appears recurrently to refer to this is spiritual or volitional essences.[7] It implies a capacity consciously to commit ourselves to a particular activity.

We have previously referred to Hahnemann's assessment of the role of volition in raising an arm. Here he asks, is it merely muscles and bones, etc. that determine this? He answers his own question by referring to the unseen will, the choice of the individual to act in such a way. It is a simple illustration but has profound implications. Throughout life we make a series of choices that affect our jobs, relationships, health and understanding, and ourselves experience the results. These, and many other instances of personal choices determining their own effects, imply our essential self-responsibility. That is, that we have a capacity for self-direction that can be increasingly understood and applied in our own situation. Such a concept is both challenging and reassuring. It is fundamental to our own sense of *self*-value. Most people prefer intelligent self-direction to imposition. A freedom to respond appropriately is preferred to passive vulnerability. Arguably, increased realization of a capacity for intelligent personal choice is an aspect of the full health which Hahnemann saw as the goal of therapy.[8]

In addition to looking at such an hierarchy of personal factors relevant to the causes of health and disease, Hahnemann refers to influences beyond the person, for instance the effects of the environment in which a patient lives. Hahnemann paid particular attention to the effects on health of living in marshy areas. He refers particularly to "intermittent diseases", such as the recurring bouts of fever due to malaria, and emphasizes the importance of the environment in their development. Even here, though, he again suggests that such environmental effects are not the only cause of diseases in people reacting to them. His opinion was that the adverse effects of the environment combined with other causes of disease, described earlier in this chapter;[9] and that all of these were liable to interact with yet another factor highly important in the development of disease. This additional factor he termed a "miasm".[10]

The term "miasm" is not widely used today and is probably now unfamiliar to most people. Briefly summarized, its former usage implied the idea that disease was due to an influential field affecting an individual patient. The definition in Wyld's *Universal English Dictionary* explains that it comes from root forms meaning a stain or a colouring and likening it to an infectious or damp mist. Such theories were popular before the discovery of micro-organisms and their part in causing disease. Miasms were regarded as an influence retained in the body of a person and capable of producing obvious disease. Hahnemann's view was that such latent traits were liable to activation either by the physical, emotional or intellectual traumas already described as possible causes of disease, or by environmental factors such as an unhealthy marsh.[11]

The idea that disease is due to the combined effects of a long-held inner and previously hidden trait, activated by more recent trauma from the environment, occupies much of Hahnemann's writing. For him, all the five levels of consciousness to which we have referred in this chapter could interact with a miasmic trait to produce disease. He even goes so far at times as to say that many acute diseases are due to transient explosions of a latent miasm.

Hahnemann's views on miasms acquire particular emphasis when he distinguishes two major types of disease, that is, acute and chronic. This is of such importance to Hahnemann's developing philosophy that it merits detailed analysis and will be the subject of the next chapter.

REFERENCES

1. *Organon* 6th Edition Paras 11, 77, 78
2. Ibid. Para. 100
3. Ibid. Paras 260, 261
4. Ibid. Para. 74
5. Ibid. Para. 225
6. Ibid. Para. 81a
7. Ibid. Paras 9–16, 269, 270
8. Ibid. Para. 9
9. Ibid. Para. 244
10. Ibid. Paras 5, 78–80
11. Ibid. Paras 81, 81a

CHAPTER IV

Acute and Chronic Diseases

FIRST WE NEED to look at these terms "acute" and "chronic". Applied in relation to diseases they denote duration of time (*chronos*). Acute diseases are relatively short-lasting episodes of illness such as measles or acute bronchitis. Chronic are those that are naturally longer-lasting, for instance rheumatoid arthritis or diabetes. Sometimes such chronic diseases show acute exacerbations of symptoms, in which case there may be talk of an acute stage of a chronic disease. An example is an acute flare-up in the severity of previously chronic and less severe rheumatoid arthritis. At times the chronic pain experienced with this illness can become markedly and quickly worse, together with an increase of the temperature and swelling of the joints as well as a decline in the general health. This type of reaction is likely to be described as an acute exacerbation of a chronic disease.

Hahnemann applied the terms in a similar way in his day. For him, too, acute implied short-lasting, chronic a longer duration of disease. But, as was his habit, Hahnemann did not stop at this relatively superficial assessment but probed more deeply into the nature of the processes involved. Even in his basic definition of the diseases that he terms acute or chronic, Hahnemann refers to the dynamic factors giving rise to them, and relates their temporal duration to the correction or persistence of vital-force changes. It is a natural development of his view that all visible disease symptoms are produced by invisible changes in the vital force.

Acute, short-lasting disease is attributed by Hahnemann to a disturbance of the vital force that is relatively quickly overcome by the body's own energies.[1] Today we might describe it as an illness to which the body's own healing process can respond in due course and restore health without necessarily needing treatment. An example would be a common cold. We might choose to try and shorten its course by treatment, but given time it resolves spontaneously. Chronic disease is a different type of process. Instead of effective reaction to and correction of the disruption, there is ineffectual opposition that fails to rectify the disturbance. Hahnemann deduces that a series of stimuli gradually disrupt the vital force in chronic disease and leave it weakened to such a degree that it no longer has the reserve needed to correct itself. He describes the vital-force resistance as "imperfect, inappropriate and ineffective".[2] Instead of the short sharp resistance that corrects the changes in acute disease, there is niggling resistance that not only fails to restore balance and reinstate the essential order, but also itself further weakens the vital force and aggravates the problem.

In other words, it becomes a vicious circle. In failing to overcome the disturbance that already exists, the ineffective resistance itself adds to the problem and feeds the disease process. We could liken it to someone with influenza insisting on getting up and working, then finding that he becomes more tired and unwell for the effort and so feels generally worse. The ineffective resistance aggravates the problem instead of overcoming it. Hahnemann describes this chain of disease, ineffective opposition to it from the vital force, further weakness and therefore a persistence and probable worsening of symptoms, as the cycle leading to chronic illness. He argues that nature therefore needs help to break this negative spiral and restore order.

In his discussions of chronic diseases Hahnemann again questions their cause in detail and considers factors as diverse as drugs and miasms. We will look first at his views on drug effects and later at miasmic influences.

Drugs such as mercury products, quinine and opium were widely used in Hahnemann's day in ways that he often criticized as inappropriate and dangerous. In his opinion such drugs were frequently applied in doses that were inadequate to overcome the diseases for which they were prescribed; and, in addition, themselves caused further weakening of the vital force. He reasoned that they set up ineffective opposition to the disease, themselves weakened the vital force and therefore aggravated the problem.[3] In short, he saw them as toxic as well as inadequate and another frequent cause of the debilitating cycle leading to chronic disease. For similar reasons he also castigated the over-use of blood-letting and purgatives.[4] These, too, he said, were often used in a manner that not only failed to rectify the disease, but also themselves further weakened the body. His comments on the adverse effects of such therapy were very blunt. Phrases such as "hostile and destructive attacks", "renewed hostile attacks of ruinous forces" occur frequently in his writings. Not surprisingly, his persistent, strongly stated arguments that such therapeutic measures commonly aggravated chronic disease, contributed to his progressive estrangement from the orthodox medical men of his day.

Although Hahnemann included such effects of abused medication in his lists of causes of chronic disease, he excluded the effects of repetitive trauma that he considered avoidable, Such effects, he said, should not be termed chronic disease in the way he applied the term.[5] He therefore excluded from his category of true chronic diseases the effects of too much food or drink, excessive mental exertion or emotional stress, prolonged lack of exercise and inappropriate housing. These effects, he argued, were due to avoidable trauma, and able to be corrected by environmental changes. Since external change could rectify these problems they were excluded from his category of chronic disease where the vital force has been weakened to such a degree that peripheral changes cannot correct its disturbance and there is need for a correctly chosen homoeopathic stimulus.

This does not imply that Hahnemann under-played the importance of such dietary, environmental and related factors for health or disease. His writings imply that he took great care over them and insisted on careful attention to their role in therapy. But in his assessment of diseases, he argues that the effects of trauma from such outside causes require similar environmental correction. By contrast, he reasons, chronic disease is determined by an inner change and requires correction by a similarly interior stimulus.

His attention to inward and hidden causal factors of chronic disease is emphasized when he looks at the role of miasms in chronic disease. In the early and middle nineteenth century, when Hahnemann was practising as a physician, miasms were considered to be a type of aura or influential force that could cause disease. The term has lapsed from use today as the concept it represented has been displaced by the discovery of bacteria and other micro-organisms associated with infection. But in Hahnemann's day it was still widely used. He accepted it and applied it in relation to the development of diseases, especially the chronic forms. He reasoned that miasms hidden within a person can be activated by the range of factors he has previously considered as causes of disease. In his opinion, the latent trait of a miasm might lie dormant in a person for much of his life, or be aroused by stimuli from physical trauma, emotional or ideological conflicts, to pro- duce obvious symptoms of a wide range of diseases.[6]

Hahnemann goes further than simply saying that miasms exist and render people vulnerable to disease. He classifies them into particular types linked to named dis- eases from which he says they have arisen. The three names he uses are syphilis, sycosis and psora, referring to the after-effects that, in his view, stemmed from syphilis, gonorrhoea and a recurrent itchy skin eruption, perhaps scabies. He reasons that certain disease patterns develop when the particular trait is activated by a contemporary stimulus. Syphilis he relates to diseases presenting with ulceration and swollen glands; sycosis with soft fleshy tumours, warty eruptions and discharges; and psora with irritating skin eruptions.[7]

These three miasmic traits, he alleges, are fundamental to the development of disease, particularly its chronic forms. He describes them as playing a major role in weakening the vital force to such a degree that the natural defences of the patient cannot correct the disorder so that the disease persists. Hence, he argues, the vital force needs the aid of a correctly prescribed antipsoric, antisyphilitic or antisycotic remedy.[8] Here again, Hahnemann deduces a theory and then applies it therapeutically.

In the sixth edition of the *Organon* Hahnemann expands his definition of psora and its effects to embrace many wide-ranging conditions. For instance, his list includes "hysteria . . . cancer . . . haemorrhoids . . . asthma . . . kidney stones . . . all kinds of pain".[9] It is very extensive and for some readers too all-embracing to be valid or useful in assessing individual disease states. But whatever we may ourselves think of the detailed application by Hahnemann of his miasm theory, it arguably plays an important role in reminding us to look for the convergence of latent, perhaps hereditary, traits, as well as recent stimuli in the evolution of disease.

An example today could be a child described as generally less well and more vulnerable to common problems such as tonsillitis and otitis media following a severe infection such as whooping cough. The earlier infection, we may deduce, left an after-effect that resulted in the child being more susceptible to other common ear and throat problems. In this situation the trait lingering from the whooping cough may be likened to the retained miasms described by Hahnemann. In homoeopathic practice the theory could be applied by treating the whooping cough effects as well as the recent symptoms.

Such theories were being deduced and written by Hahnemann long before Pasteur discovered bacteria, and later researchers found the micro-organisms associated with syphilis, gonorrhoea and scabies. In the light of such disclosures, and the growth of scientific medicine that followed them, Hahnemann's theories may at first appear out-dated and of historical interest only. On closer review, however, his deductions can be seen to anticipate the bacterial theories to be evolved later. For instance, an extract of Hahnemann's writings on cholera, quoted by his biographer Haehl, reads, "The cholera miasm . . . probably consists of a murderous organism, undetected to our senses, which attaches itself to a man's skin, hair etc."[10] A similar idea is expressed in the *Organon* when Hahnemann writes on epidemic diseases such as measles and smallpox. His references to a causal agent are translated as "an unvarying infectious agent",[11] or "a contagious principle that always remains the same".[12] His thoughts here can be seen as a bridge between the old idea of an ill-defined miasmic vapour contributing to disease and the subsequent discovery of precise pathogenic organisms. It appears that to Hahnemann the "murderous organism" or "infectious agent" that he anticipates, is a focal expression of the miasmic force. Again, it is a polarized assessment with the visible aspect, although only seen with a microscope, giving evidence of the unseen, influential field.

Such an opinion can be supported by the scientific insights now available. We know today that micro-organisms such as bacteria, viruses and the cholera vibrio are important factors in causing disease. We know, too, that even such defined organisms are energy phenomena. Seen in this way, both the theory of pathogenic organisms and the ideas of influential force fields have their place in an assessment of the causes of disease.

Over the years, since Hahnemann developed his views on miasms, there has been a lot of discussion among homoeo-paths concerning the way in which these causes of disease are transmitted. Many have assumed that when Hahnemann, writing on psora, refers to the "gradual transmission and incredible development of this ancient contagion, for hundreds of generations and through millions of human organisms", he is implying a hereditary trait.[13] Others have said that he is still referring to skin contact passing the trait on, so that it is acquired after birth. Some translators of the *Organon* appear to interpret Hahnemann's writings as allowing for both possibilities.[14] The debate continues. But, either way, Hahnemann's references to miasms imply a predisposition to disease operating within a person. Whether it is inherited pre-birth or acquired by contact shortly post-birth, it remains within the individual body and, he argues, is liable to reactivation by other stimuli acquired in time, with the two together producing obvious disease.[15]

The idea of a latent trait activated by a further stimulus is an interesting one that is worth looking at more closely. It is widely acknowledged today that some diseases are due to a combination of consciously recognized recent traumas and unconscious or hidden factors, possibly hereditary. One example is the precipitation by recent environmental factors of a previously latent hereditary trait predisposing to peptic ulceration. These ideas are easier to consider if we remember that all aspects of the human body, including its physical structures, are dynamic. They are patterns of energy able to retain imprints of past experiences, including trauma and infection. A retained trace of an old disorder may conjoin with a recent disturbance to produce a particular pattern of disease in the present.

The miasmic traits, which Hahnemann describes as hidden until they are activated to produce obvious symptoms, may also be thought of as relics of ancestral unsatisfied drive or disease sufficiently disruptive to produce a lasting imprint. The theories on protoplasmic inheritance remind us that personal characteristics can be passed from generation to generation. Is it not possible that part of this inheritance can also be the remembered frustrations or diseases experienced with sufficient intensity in an individual lifetime to leave their mark on the personal protoplasm? And is it not reasonable then to go a stage further and suggest that this may be another aspect of the miasmic trait that Hahnemann argues is prone to reactivation in the development of disease in the present? Overt disease can be an expression of personal vectors of which we are not individually aware but which remain operant within our organism and influence its response to a wide range of environmental stimuli, including bacteria, viruses and other agents.

Hahnemann set high standards for his own work, for the colleagues who joined him in the early development of homoeopathic practice, and for those of us continuing such commitments today. The investigation of such a wide range of possible causes of diseases and similarly careful evaluation of their effects, implies the need for a very careful review of the case histories presented by people seeking homoeopathic treatment. Clearly a review that is both precise and comprehensive is required if it is to investigate hints of lingering traces of disturbance predisposing to disease in the present, recent events provoking their emergence, after effects of other therapies, and details of the symptoms arising from the conjoined effects of such stimuli. Hence Hahnemann's precise instructions on how to assess a patient's report.

REFERENCES

1. *Organon* 6th Edition   Para. 72
2. Ibid.   Para. 72
3. Ibid.   Para. 74
4. Ibid.   Paras 74a, 75, 76 Introduction
5. Ibid.   Para. 77
6. Ibid.   Paras 78, 78a, 81a
7. Ibid.   Paras 79, 80, 204, 206
8. Ibid.   Paras 80a, 204
9. Ibid.   Para. 80
10. *Samuel Hahnemann. His Life and Work*.   Haehl Ch. 15
11. *Organon* 6th Edition   Para. 100 trans. Künzli, Naudé and Pendleton
12. *Organon* 6th Edition   Para. 100

trans. Dudgeon and Boericke

13. *Organon* 6th Edition   Para. 81
    trans. Künzli, Naudé and

Pendleton

14. Ibid.   Para. 78a

15. *Organon* 6th Edition   Para. 78a

CHAPTER V

Hahnemann's Advice on Case-History Taking

FUNDAMENTAL TO HAHNEMANN's advice on how to assess
reports of disease in order to prescribe are two basic themes
previously noted in this study. That is, that the symptoms
presented are always individual or unique to that person at
that stage in his or her life, and that they are always the
outward, visible signs of inward, unseen dynamics. In
practice this implies the need always to be alert for the
unexpected and to remember that all symptoms are the
relatively superficial aspects of disease processes and need
careful evaluation if we are to understand their hidden
determinants. Hahnemann's application of such ideals led
him to investigate events such as physical injury, bereavement or personal insult that may have been related to the
onset of symptoms, as well as the precise details of their effects.

Several paragraphs of the *Organon* are particularly concerned with the assessment of data presented by patients.[1]
Right at the beginning of his instructions Hahnemann
emphasizes the particular importance of physical symptoms, mood changes or any other features that are a definite
contrast to a person's previous state. If we are assessing the
process occurring at a particular time, the changes from a
prior state are especially significant. This may appear to be
stating the obvious, but it is a useful reminder to look for the
process new to a given moment and not to assume that an
individual's personality and physiology have been previously established, then continued as a "constitution" that
may need treatment throughout his life.

I emphasize this point because it is apparent from the
discussions that follow many meetings on homoeopathy,
that the writings of James Tyler Kent (an American doctor

who practiced homoeopathy in the late nineteenth and early twentieth century) have often been assumed to imply that there is an individual "constitutional" picture presented by a person throughout his life. It is then suggested that such a profile can be a basis for prescribing a homoeopathic remedy. Whether or not this is a correct interpretation of Kent's writings is not a subject we need to pursue here. But it is certainly not Hahnemann's view. He draws attention to the importance of recent changes in a patient's account of his symptoms as a guide to assessing his present health or disease. This does not discount the need also to observe processes that are relatively unchanged for him and part of his present assessment. It is simply stating a useful parameter for assessing the process now presented by a patient seeking help.

In order to collect as clear a picture as possible of all such changes, Hahnemann advises noting first the patient's reports of his symptoms, next what the relatives say has happened, and thirdly the physician's own observations.[2] The physician's observations should include detailed questioning to clarify the reports given, as well as findings from his examinations of the patient. In all of these stages we see again that Hahnemann is looking for evidence of what the patient is experiencing, both physically and in the less obvious aspects, as well as for clues about the causes of such effects. He advises noting with meticulous care the symptoms reported and asking appropriate, but not leading, questions where clarification is needed. His attention to detail includes reference to the exact nature of any physical changes reported; their context, or the general health of the patient; his use of other therapies or drugs; his housing and family background. We will take a closer look at this.

The particular symptoms are usually the major concern of the patient, and also the first aspect of this wide and detailed review that he is likely to present. Hahnemann advocates taking careful notes of such reports, paying particular attention to the precise form, timing, quality and intensity of symptoms, and any event that appears related to their onset or deterioration. For instance, in relation to bowel symptoms he advises asking about the frequency of stools; their nature and any accompaniment such as mucus; their colour; any pain when they are passed, and if so its precise form; and any circumstances that may appear to have caused the changes.[3]

In the years since Hahnemann made such recommendations many homoeopaths have devised particular schemes to assist the pursuit of this aim. A term used by many prescribers refers to the "modalities" of symptoms. These are particular circumstances that may provoke changes in the symptoms patients report. Examples are changes of posture, physical rest or movement, diet, time of day, being in company or alone, changes in the weather. For instance, a homoeopathic prescriber will note a particular woman's headache is worse when the head is moved, often comes on about 11 a.m. and is intensified by drinking coffee, or if visitors arrive and try to offer help. Such details, known as modalities, can be a great help for building up the profile needed for detailed homoeopathic prescribing.

In his review of the general state of the patient, we might call it the context of the particular symptoms, Hahnemann advises noting such features as the overall state of physical health; the mood or temperament; dietary and climatic likes and dislikes; the quality, duration of, and position for, sleeping; the patterns of exercise and rest; and sexual habits. Here again, as well as observing these features at a given moment, note is taken of how they vary with changing circumstances.[4] In other words, the modalities are again noted for the general features in a manner similar to that used in relation to the particular symptoms. A prescriber following this approach today would therefore ask about the responses of the patient himself to such variables as the time of day or night, the season of the year, exercise or rest, diet, weather, company or solitude, etc.

Patients often volunteer such information and distinguish

between changes in their general responses as opposed to their particular symptoms. An instance is a patient with rheumatoid arthritis who reports that her joints feel worse in a cold sea breeze, but she loves it and feels generally better for it.

Such general responses include the psychological features of the patient's overall presentation. Here again, Hahnemann looks for both the easily recognized and the less obvious data. Emotional symptoms are obvious when a patient's main complaint is of anxiety or depression. They can be similarly obvious in association with major physical symptoms. For instance, someone with influenza or a broken leg may also readily admit to feeling depressed. But in many other disease states patients try to hide such reactions. This may be because they regard admission of anxiety or depression as personal weakness, morally wrong, anti-social or not permitted by a British stiff upper lip. Conversely some people will give exaggerated reports of symptoms and their personal reactions to them. All such reactions are part of the patient's situation and, Hahnemann reminds us, to be examined with care.[5]

Closely related to such effects are changes with an emphasis on thought processes. Sometimes it is debatable whether anxious thoughts are a cause of, or are caused by, disease. But either way they are commonly a major part of a disease process. As Hahnemann reminds us, worry about family matters, business stress, questions about long-held beliefs or morals, etc. often play a major role in a patient's disease. Many patients try to ignore or repress such conflicts and pretend they are not worried. But this only makes matters even worse as the inheld tensions remain and the effort of repressing them places yet more demands on a patient's energy reserves. Such repression is often a result of conditioning that patients have received in their early years teaching that it is "wrong" to show such worry, voice personal conflicts, or express anxieties openly. Hahnemann's references to such effects imply first his understanding of their possible role in the development of disease processes, and second his awareness that they can easily lead to distortion or denial of reported symptoms.[6] It is now approximately 130 years since Hahnemann died. In that time many other thinkers have similarly described the way in which restrictive thought-patterns contribute to disease. In recent years many researchers have supported such insight by showing that psychological states change body chemistry and directly affect the physical symptoms, proving again that the mind–body are aspects of a continuum where the various levels of function interact all the time. Hahnemann implied his understanding of such a non-dualistic assessment of disease long before its scientific backing was discovered. It is evident in his writings on case-history taking, when he advises noting not only what patients say, but how they say it, their manner of presentation and speech, their appearance, temperament and posture;[7] all of which are further guides to these less obvious but similarly important hidden psychological processes.

For instance, two women may go to a doctor complaining of painful periods, known technically as dysmenorrhoea. They may report apparently similar symptoms of painful lower abdominal cramps, nausea and tiredness. But if one is irritable, chilly and sweaty and not wanting sympathy, while the other is warm blooded, dry skinned and craving sympathy, they clearly have different chemistry involved and individual prescribing needs.

After such a careful review of patients' reported symptoms, Hahnemann turns his attention to their housing and other regular aspects of their daily routine. He observes that housing conditions, abuse of drugs, too much or too little exercise, sleep, food or drink, as well as sexual licence or repression can strongly influence the course of a disease.[8] Hence his advice that due attention needs to be paid to all of these factors in taking a patient's case history. He was concerned to clarify any association between such factors and the onset, prolonging, change or relief of any symptoms.

Another aspect of a patient's medical history considered important for prescribing today concerns familiar disease patterns. It is generally acknowledged, now, that hereditary traits can play an important part in the development of many disease states. Although Hahnemann does not refer to this directly in the paragraphs of the *Organon* specifically concerned with case-history taking, he implies its import-ance in other sections. For instance, very early in the *Organon* he refers to the need when assessing a patient's medical problems to note his family background.[9] Other references to possible hereditary factors to be noted are seen by some homoeopaths in Hahnemann's many references to the miasms discussed in the previous chapter. As noted there, Hahnemann deduced that these retained effects of prior diseases may lie dormant for many years until they are activated by a recent stimulus to produce obvious symp-toms.

Such detailed case-history taking was advocated by Hahnemann for all diseases, especially for those of a chronic nature. Even for assessing epidemic diseases Hahnemann requires similar attention to individual prescribing needs. He argues that collecting the composite details from several patients is important for an assessment of a particular epidemic reaction.[10] Applying such advice today means noting in an outbreak of influenza features such as a raised temperature, backache, headache and sore throat shown by many patients, individual features such as particular sweat-ing patterns and minimal thirst shown by a few of the patients, and summating all these data to select a remedy appropriate to the epidemic process.

For all stages of such assessments Hahnemann requires particular standards and methods of approach from the physician. Prominent in his list is impartiality.[11] That is, the avoidance of any bias by the prescriber from his own concerns, and not letting himself be influenced by prejudice shown by relatives. This does not imply discounting rela-tives' reports of a patient's symptoms. It is clear that

Hahnemann welcomed these as additional aids for assessing individual patients.[12] It is simply a practical reminder not to be over influenced by what relatives say. For the physician himself, it also means not putting words into patients' mouths or trying to lead them to answers that will fit in with quick assessments made on an initial meeting.

Such avoidance of bias is the negative aspect in the physician's approach. The positive is to be ready for the unexpected. This is clearly a requisite when there is an emphasis on the individuality of disease. Every patient is a unique being, his case history is therefore peculiar to him and we are not to assume that set patterns of symptoms will be presented. If we anticipate answers and load questions to get the expected replies, or go even further and suggest to patients what we think they are experiencing, we are assuming that they are reacting like people we have known before and paying less attention to the uniqueness of their situation.

Such detailed questioning of patients and other relevant people is only a first stage in the assessment. Hahnemann also emphasized the value of a thorough medical examination in which the physician's observations are added to the developing profile needed for homoeopathic prescribing.[13] We need here to recall the era in which Hahnemann was working. A medical examination in his day obviously lacked the refined diagnostic aids now available. Some people argue that this made physicians such as Hahnemann more astute observers themselves and less reliant on technological aids.

Today, however, we need to consider the role of additional investigations such as blood tests, X-rays, and other scientific health checks. Homoeopathic doctors frequently advise their use if they are appropriate to help understand a disease. Obviously they have an important role in modern medicine. The results of such investigations are added to the findings, or physical signs, noted on examination of a patient, and all of these data are appended to the reported symptoms. The terminology of today therefore distinguishes

54

between the "signs" of disease found by doctors, and the "symptoms" initially reported by patients. Reading translations of Hahnemann's writings today could therefore suggest that he regarded patients' reports of symptoms as the primary guides for homoeopathic prescribing and that even today special physical tests need not be necessary. On careful reading, however, we note that Hahnemann's use of the term "symptoms" applies to all detectable after-effects of hidden causes of diseases.[14] We may therefore argue that findings from a careful physical examination and results of similarly detailed laboratory tests which also yield measurable evidence of hidden disease processes, may also be termed "symptoms". Seen in this way the use, in homoeopathic prescribing today, of such measurements of disease-effects may be seen as not inconsistent with Hahnemann's ideals.

For all the data obtained, Hahnemann insists on careful, well ordered note-taking,[15] clearly essential if so many lines of questioning are to be pursued and then integrated into an individual profile. All of this is intended to assist a clear assessment by both the patient and the prescriber of the individual process. It continually refers to the individuality of the patient, and to the awareness that his particular symptoms are the relatively superficial evidence of a dynamic process relevant to his whole person.

When people consult a homoeopathic doctor for the first time they often express surprise at some of the questions asked and comment that they have not previously considered their reactions in sufficient detail to give an answer. The questioning can often usefully provoke people to assess their personal responses more accurately and to give answers that have a dual purpose. The first and obvious use is to aid selection of a homoeopathic stimulus in hopes of removing unpleasant symptoms. The second is to increase self-knowledge through a more precise assessment of what is happening. If this process is followed with the care and precision advocated by Hahnemann, both the prescriber and the patient will have a better understanding of the situation.

Such a growth of insight is an important implication of the similia therapy advocated by Hahnemann. The increase of insight concerning the nature and causes of disease is an essential step towards realizing personal control of health, in all its aspects. It is often said that adequate recognition of a problem is at least half way to overcoming it. Less than this is like trying to remove a splinter without first seeing where it is. One implication of the similia principle is that it enhances a patient's recognition of what is happening to him. That is, it increases personal consciousness of body processes and makes way for the next step, the redirection or change of body functions.

Such a comment on the implications of the similia concept is merely an introduction to a fundamental principle of homoeopathy. We will examine it further in the next chapter.

REFERENCES

1. *Organon* 6th Edition   Paras 83–103
2. Ibid.   Para. 84
3. Ibid.   Paras 86, 89, 89a, 93, 94
4. Ibid.   Para. 88
5. Ibid.   Paras 96–98
6. Ibid.   Para. 93
7. Ibid.   Paras 90, 90a
8. Ibid.   Paras 93, 94
9. Ibid.   Para. 5
10. Ibid.   Paras 101, 102
11. Ibid.   Para. 83
12. Ibid.   Paras 84, 85, 98
13. Ibid.   Paras 84, 90, 90a
14. Ibid.   Paras 14, 17
15. Ibid.   Paras 83–87

CHAPTER VI

Similar, Palliative and Allopathic Effects

HAHNEMANN'S CONCEPT OF the therapeutic similia required for an effective and thorough treatment of disease is often summarized by his own Latin phrase, "Similia similibus curentur", or by its translation "let likes be treated by likes". These are both brief descriptions attempting to simplify a principle with far-reaching and provocative implications. The practical application, using appropriately minute doses of agents that can cause symptoms to treat similar effects when they occur in the course of a disease, was hinted at by Hippocrates long before Hahnemann's relatively recent restatement of it. Using an extract of onion to treat a particular form of a common cold is an easily quoted example of an application which has steadily progressed from very early civilizations, through Hahnemann's era, to contemporary medicine. Like many aspects of daily experience, we can see it at this relatively superficial level or probe its implications.

One way of starting such probing is to begin by considering what similia are not. It is sometimes apparent in discussions of homoeopathy today that some people interpret the similia concept as meaning a mimicry of common disease symptoms. They suggest, like some of the early Greek philosophers, that discharges from the body such as sweating, diarrhoea or vomiting are nature's way of clearing diseases and are to be encouraged. They then assume that the similia of homoeopathy imply encouraging these common symptoms in order to discharge diseases. Hahnemann's writings strongly refute such a superficial interpretation. Many times he emphatically denounces the attempts by many of his contemporary physicians to treat disease by provoking symptoms like sweating, vomiting, diarrhoea and blood-letting. He argues that symptoms are the body's automatic "unreasoned" reactions to disease and that to mimic or provoke them further, not only does not help the defence process, but actually impedes it. Such mimicry of symptoms already present, he deduces, aggravates an initial and first-stage reaction in disease, further weakens the body, and makes it more difficult for the "healing art" to produce an appropriate second-stage correction.[1]

In more detail, Hahnemann's argument is that there are two stages in disease and healing, termed by him primary and secondary reactions. The primary reaction is the initial effect produced in response to injury, infection, mental or other trauma. The secondary reaction is the body's adjustment or healing process. That is, the reaction to restore a healthy balance.[2] He says therefore that aiming to mimic or increase the primary reaction is aggravating the situation and making it even harder for an effective secondary or restoring action by the vital force. A simple example is to compare the initial or primary reaction to the blood loss that occurs when a blood vessel is cut. The corrective secondary action includes the contraction of the vessel and blood clotting to stem the loss. Encouraging bleeding before the correction can occur is only adding to the problems. Hence, Hahnemann argues, the need is to stimulate and reinforce the body's counteraction to the disease and not to mimic its preliminary effects.

The simillimum (a specific application of the similia principle) of Hahnemann therefore differs from an exaggeration of the usual effects of disease in two ways. First, it is not an agent that is designed necessarily to provoke more sweating, purging or other exudates in hopes of mimicking common disease symptoms and expelling the causes of the problem. Its apparently pathological effects, the symptoms it is capable of producing if taken by healthy volunteers, are intended to match the particular symptoms of the individual disease process as closely as possible. At times this may include a change of bowel habit, when for instance arsenicum extracts are used in the treatment of gastroenteritis.[3] But increased bowel activity need not be a feature of many other homoeopathic similia.

Secondly, the intention behind a homoeopathic simillimum is the provocation of the second stage or counteraction to the disease and not merely the primary or initial symptoms, even if these include diarrhoea, sweating, etc. It is intended to stimulate the counteraction more than the initial symptomatic effect. In other words, the simillimum is an attempt to increase the reaction against the disease and is certainly not mere mimicry of symptoms.[4]

The simillimum advocated by Hahnemann is therefore a stimulus intended to arouse an appropriate response to counteract particular disease symptoms. From his observations of the body's responses to individual medicines, Hahnemann deduced that their primary action was individual and characteristic in form and duration. He even calls it "a law" of nature, saying that through careful experiment the precise primary effects of particular medicinal agents can be observed and recorded.[5] As a result of this highly individual initial disturbance, he reasoned, the vital force produced a counteraction, or secondary action, in an attempt to restore stability in the organism. The primary change he describes as a passive effect due to the action of the medicine; the secondary as an active response.

Hahnemann deduced his theories from observations of body responses to various stimuli commonly encountered. For example, he observes that a man warmed by too much wine (primary action) is likely later on to feel chilly as the counteraction, or hangover, develops (secondary action). Or, with drug effects, experiencing heightened liveliness from drinking a lot of coffee (primary effect), may be followed by drowsiness and tiredness (secondary effect) unless the coffee intake is repeated.[6] We could illustrate it in another way be saying that the primary effect is like the displacement of water as a ball is dropped into it, the secondary change is the reaction by the water itself so that the ball is pushed on to the surface and floats.

Hahnemann applies his understanding of primary and secondary responses to therapeutic stimulation by "similia" medicines and the contrasting hazards of "palliatives" and "contraria".[7] These three terms were used commonly by Hahnemann in describing the types of therapy he saw practised. The simillimum, as we have noted many times, implies an agent capable of provoking symptoms that closely resemble those of the original disease for which treatment is sought. The palliative is its opposite. It is an agent capable of producing an immediate opposite effect to the disease and hopefully therefore of directly masking the original symptoms.[8] A common example is the use of pain-relieving tablets, technically known as "analgesics". The third type of treatment, the contraria or allopathy, is a type of distraction. It neither mimics nor directly opposes the previous symptoms but instead arouses a different type of vital force reaction that is "neither similar nor opposite but completely heterogeneous". Such drugs, Hahnemann observed, were often prescribed because they had appeared useful for treatment previously, although they were neither similars or palliatives and therefore lacked a direct relationship to the specific symptoms of a particular disease process. He describes them as selected by "conjecture" and "intended to divert sickness to other parts".[9]

When Hahnemann looks in detail at the effects of palliatives he is slightly less dismissive of their use than he is of allopathic drugs. The primary action of the palliative drug, he observes, directly opposes the prior symptoms and so quickly affords relief.[10] He also admits that there are occasions when such therapeutic measures may be vital. Resuscitation after choking or near-drowning is one of the examples he cites when sudden stimulation may be required from a primary action to oppose the trauma effects.[11]

But whilst he admits that the contrary stimulus may be important to therapy in such an emergency, he also strongly warns against its inappropriate use in other situations. His observations, and then his deductions concerning primary and secondary actions, told him that after the initial relief from palliative stimuli there followed a worsening of the symptoms. He cites the particular example of pain relief, pointing out that in diseases where pain continues a long time the dose of an analgesic needs increasing with its repetition.[12] This is well known today. A common example is the use of morphine derivatives for long-lasting pain. A continuing use over several weeks usually leads to the need for increasing doses to sustain a similar level of pain control. It is known technically as "tolerance". Hahnemann explains this by reasoning that the primary action of the pain reliever directly opposes the pain symptoms and at first brings relief. But, after this, the secondary reaction of the vital force against this relieving primary change brings an intensification of the original state, and therefore provokes more pain and the need for increasing doses of the medicine. These larger doses of medicine, he argues, in turn lead to a proportional increase in the secondary intensification of the pain and so on. It therefore becomes a vicious circle with medicines apparently helpful in their initial stages leading to more problems in the longer term.

The need to discriminate between a helpful use of palliatives and an unhelpful provocation of chronic diseases is a difficulty still faced today. Patients with short-term severe pain may well recover quickly both from the illness and from the analgesics used to treat it. A common example is relief of post-operative pain. Here the course of treatment is so short that progressive tolerance of drugs due to increasing secondary reactions to their initial effects, and therefore a need for larger doses of medicines, are not likely to be seen. The problem is more difficult with long-term painful disease. Humanitarian concern to relieve pain and offer appropriate aids to ensure rest required for repair of body structures, even though it requires increasing doses of analgesics, often overrides concern about secondary reactions aggravating the underlying process. The two extremes of short-lasting post-operative states and long-term chronic disease may be stark enough to distinguish. The intermediate ground is much more difficult. It can be a dilemma both for prescribers and patients.

As well as considering palliatives Hahnemann also probes the details of responses to allopathic drugs, and he again employs his understanding of primary and secondary reactions to stimuli. As we briefly noted earlier he uses the term allopathic to refer to a drug stimulus, the primary action of which was neither a simillimum nor a directly opposing palliative for the original disease. He argues firmly against the use of such medicines saying they only afford apparent relief at times by a type of distraction from the previous disease pattern. They then leave the original disease unchanged or at times also append their own ongoing effects, making matters even worse for the patient.[13]

It is relevant here to emphasize how Hahnemann uses the term allopathic in relation to medicines, as the term is often applied less precisely today. He did not use it for every medicine that was not homoeopathic. He applied it strictly to drugs with an effect dissimilar but not opposite to a previously existing disease for which a medicine is required. He deduced that if this was stronger than that particular disease it could temporarily become the dominant effect on the vital force. Hence while its action lasted the disease pattern was veiled for a time but not actually changed. As the drug effect receded the disease reappeared.

In his discussions of these processes and in the examples cited Hahnemann refers to interactions between differing natural diseases, or natural disease processes, and the effects of medicinal stimuli that he sometimes terms medicinal diseases.[14] This argument is easier to follow if we recall that Hahnemann regarded all disease processes, whether infectious or traumatic in origin, and the results of medicinal stimuli, as produced by changes in the vital force. He therefore refers to both disease/disease, or disease/medicine interactions when he refers to the results of homoeopathic, palliative and allopathic stimuli, particularly in his examples of allopathic stimuli from other natural diseases or medicines appearing briefly to displace a previous malady so that it seems temporarily relieved while the new one takes over. He observed, for instance, children with epilepsy whose seizures remitted while they had a scalp infection known as *tinea capitis*, but recurred as the infection cleared.[15] This is one type of response Hahnemann reports from allopathic stimuli. He also comments on two more.

One is no effect at all if the medicinal stimulus is the same strength or weaker than the original. Here the prior disturbance remains relatively unchanged. The new medicinal effect is repelled and the previous symptom picture persists. One of Hahnemann's examples of this effect was the failure of smallpox vaccination, as used in his day, to take in children already suffering from rickets. He reasons that the prior disease state was of such strength that it masked any reaction to the second stimulus.[16]

His other possibility is the joining together of medicinal effects and disease processes, particularly likely if the second stimulus, the medicine, is repeated for a long time. The original disturbance and the effects of the medicine then converge in a new, more complex disease. His example is the combined effects of two diseases such as measles and smallpox which, he claims, he occasionally saw existing together at the same time in a patient. Or, the combined effects of a disease and a drug inappropriate for its complexities. Hahnemann observed that such combined effects of two diseases, or the combination of a disease and unsuitable drugs, could produce more complex derangements of the vital force and associated symptoms.[17] Pursuing this thought in the Introduction to the *Organon*, he deduces that old-school physicians prescribing nothing more than lightly flavoured water were more likely to approach the age-old therapeutic ideal of "above all, do no harm".

Such hazards from allopathic or palliative drugs are

contrasted by Hahnemann with the advantages of a therapeutic simillimum. He again applies his observations of primary and secondary actions. The primary action of the simillimum is the provocation by the medicinal agent of symptoms that closely resemble those already occurring in the disease. He describes it as similar to and stronger than the original disease process and therefore able to mask it. This new medicinal disease, Hahnemann deduces, is short-lasting for two reasons. Its own dynamism declines naturally faster than the previous disease process would have done. The medicinal stimulus also provokes a counter-action by the vital force against itself.[18] Both of these factors contribute to the release of the vital force from the previous disturbance so that health is restored.

Hahnemann's theories of primary and secondary reactions therefore explain his observations concerning the differing effects of palliative, allopathic and homoeopathic stimuli. The palliative briefly eases but then aggravates a prior disease. The allopathic medicine may briefly distract from it for a time but then leaves the original disturbance and symptoms unchecked. Only the simillimum provokes the appropriate secondary action required to remove the disease.

Such theories concerning the effects of medicinal stimuli again indicate Hahnemann's persistent drive to understand the polarized aspects of medical phenomena. He saw gross effects and sought to look through them to their less obvious causes. To Hahnemann, the essential feature in a simillimum was its capacity, not only to provoke the visible primary effect of symptoms similar to the existing disease, but its ability then to arouse the unseen secondary reaction of the vital force. This, he argues recurrently, is the response that is essential for thorough correction of a disease process. It shows again his determination to pursue simultaneously insights into both aspects of the polarity of human consciousness. That is, the easily seen gross effects and their less easily recognized but equally important unseen dynamics. Hence his discussion of therapeutic similia is far more detailed than a mere recital of symptoms which correspond with observed effects of medicines. His concern is also for an insight into their causes.

Such concern is not an "empty speculation" as dismissed by Hahnemann in the Preface to the second edition of the *Organon*. Instead it is careful deduction based on equally careful observation of gross organic effects.

Hahnemann's use of similars correlates with his cardinal ideal of increasing Self-knowledge through observing disease and its treatment. The homoeopathic stimulus is an intentional restatement of a condition already present in an individual. Such a repetition is one way of heightening the individual consciousness of the process. It is fundamentally different from either a palliative opposing stimulus or an allopathic diversion. Both of these in effect have a suppressive action. They apparently bring relief of a problem by veiling or reducing its expression, and can therefore be described as suppressive. In contrast to this, the homoeopathic stimulus increases both the primary awareness of the problem and the secondary action to overcome it. Hence, it may be argued, the homoeopathic process works through increasing individual awareness of the problem and the activity required to correct it.

Hahnemann's observations on the nature of disease and how to understand it in order to remove it thoroughly, are an example of the reflection he advised for all medical problems and the therapies applied for them. One of his criticisms of many of his medical contemporaries concerned their lack of thorough reflection on their work with patients. He even attributes their failure to discover homoeopathy to their lack of such careful observation.[19] For Hahnemann, thorough observation and deduction of processes exhibited in diseases and their treatment was essential to his progressive understanding of a rational therapeutic system.

The six editions of the *Organon*, as well as several other major works, are evidence of his personal continuing assessment of these dynamic processes. They show how he continued to reflect on his work, deduce a rationale and then apply it in an evolving therapy.

Such continuing reappraisal was applied by Hahnemann to medicines and their effects as well as to disease processes. Earlier chapters have referred particularly to his observations on diseases and an ideal therapeutic process. The next three chapters will consider his understanding of how to test, develop and present the medicines needed for effective practice.

REFERENCES

1. *Organon* 4th Edition   Preface, *Organon* 6th Edition Para. 22a
2. *Organon* 6th Edition   Paras 63–65
3. Ibid.   Paras 24–27, 34
4. Ibid.   Paras 22, 22a
5. Ibid.   Paras 32, 33, 111
6. Ibid.   Para. 65
7. Ibid.   Paras 23, 52–59
8. Ibid.   Paras 56–59
9. Ibid.   Paras 22a, 54, 55
10. Ibid.   Paras 22, 56–60
11. Ibid.   Para. 67a
12. Ibid.   Paras 59–61, 69
13. Ibid.   Paras 38, 39, 74, 75
14. Ibid.   Paras 36–46
15. Ibid.   Para. 38
16. Ibid.   Para. 36
17. Ibid.   Paras 40–42
18. Ibid.   Paras 24–29, 43–45, 63–66
19. Ibid.   Para. 61

CHAPTER VII

Provings of Homoeopathic Medicines

WE MIGHT EXPECT Hahnemann's discussions of the medicines employed in homoeopathy to begin with a review of the sources from which they are obtained. But in the *Organon* he pays little attention to this. A few are named when he uses case reports to illustrate the principles involved and emphasizes the importance of using accurately named specimens that are as fresh as possible, or carefully preserved if coming from abroad. But in general his discussions in the *Organon* are more concerned with the nature of homoeopathic medicines and how to prepare and preserve continuing supplies. The preparation of medicines is itself a large subject and will be considered in a later chapter. Before that, we will look at Hahnemann's ideas on the nature of the medicines and how to demonstrate their effects in a test situation prior to applying them in therapy.

Visible effects of disease, Hahnemann has deduced, are due to unseen changes in the "vital force". Similarly, for medicines, he argues that their hidden dynamism determines the characteristic effects seen in people who take them. His aim in testing medicines is therefore to produce a picture of the visible effects of these invisible energies that is as accurate as possible.

We know from other works by Hahnemann, as well as from his biographers, that his personal investigations of homoeopathy began around 1791 when he took cinchona in order personally to test its effect. It was the first of many similar experiments in which Hahnemann, his family and his colleagues, personally took medicinal agents to observe details of their action. Such experiments were intended to prove the effects the agents could produce in human beings

67

and were therefore known as "provings". The testers subsequently became known as "provers". Hahnemann's idea was that if healthy, trustworthy and conscientious people, standards he set for his provers, took medicines and carefully recorded their effects, this would produce accurate data suitable for application in prescribing for disease.[1] That provers should be as healthy as possible was particularly important to Hahnemann. He reasoned that testing medicines on healthy volunteers reduced the distortion of results that would occur if obvious disease symptoms existed before a person began a proving.[2]

Hahnemann's theory was that the visible form of a medicine is a vehicle for the unseen energies essential to it. For this unseen factor he used terms subsequently translated "spirit-like essence"[3] or "conceptual essence".[4] The experimental provings are intended to show the gross effects that these subtle energies hidden within the medicine can produce. He goes a stage further when he deduces that these essential and unseen energies are able to interact suitably with the dynamic causes of disease and provoke the changes required for healing. In other words, he is saying that experimental provings demonstrate the effects of energies hidden within the medicines and able to interact appropriately with the disturbed vital force, similarly hidden within a person, and restore health.

Clearly, the change required to produce healing will need to be specific to that particular disease. This brings us again to the similia principle fundamental to Hahnemann's thought and discussed in the previous chapter. As we noted there, it states that only an agent capable of provoking a process similar to that occurring in the disease will stimulate the corresponding reaction against itself, therefore against the disease as well, and lead to healing. Provings have therefore been carried out to clarify the changes in health an individual medicine can produce, so that these can be matched with the details of symptoms in a particular disease and then applied in treatment.[5]

Many times Hahnemann claims that he is the first person in the history of the human race to deduce that medicines can be tested in this way on healthy volunteers in order to clarify the effects they can produce, and then subsequently use these for treating other people with diseases that present a similar symptom picture. It is a principle that has appealed to many people since then, one of its major advantages being the testing of medicines in human beings. Whatever our individual ethical view about testing medicines on animals, there is always the practical question of whether data produced in this way are necessarily accurate for the human species. It is a difficulty Hahnemann avoids by his insistence on testing medicines on human volunteers.

Although Hahnemann has avoided that particular difficulty others remain. Testing medicines on human beings presents other practical problems. One of the first to be mentioned nowadays will probably be the placebo response. This is a change produced by expectation of an effect. An example occurred in an experimental proving done with approximately 50 volunteers in north-west England in the late 1970s. The proving was set to run for three months. No one in the trial knew the distribution, which was placebo (a non-medicated tablet resembling the medicated form) for all provers in the first month; and either placebo or medicated tablets, one month of each in the second and third months. The effects reported in the first month far exceeded those in the rest of the trial period. They ranged from an irritant facial skin eruption or a "sudden collapse" on the kitchen floor to multiple reports of cold-type symptoms. The apparent effects from medicated tablets were much less dramatic.

To be fair to Hahnemann we have to acknowledge that the placebo effect had not been generally recognized in his day. Consequently it would be hard to blame him for not apparently taking it into account when he gives his instructions on how to do provings. Hahnemann's personal stance is, in fact, quite the reverse of allowing for placebo effects. He argues firmly that any change in health produced by a medicine in a proving is an effect of that medicine. In his opinion even idiosyncratic reactions appearing in only a few individuals, and not shown by other members of a group of provers, are still effects of that medicine and to be included in the reports of results.[6] It is a stance many would challenge today when we are more aware that personal psychology can lead people to react strongly to stimulation in ways highly individual to their own state. Consequently when provings are now planned great care is taken to try and reduce the impact of placebo responses on the results.

Although Hahnemann made no allowance for possible placebo effects in provings, the rigorous care which he applied to other aspects of these experiments is evidenced in his detailed and precise instructions on their conduct. The data he collected were of fundamental importance to his developing homoeopathic practice. Although he also used data from toxicology to augment his materia medica,[7] provings remained a cornerstone of his work. Consequently his instructions to provers were extremely careful, supporting his intention to demonstrate details of the gross organic and psychological effects that could be produced in human beings by the subtle, hidden energies of the medicine.

Hahnemann refers to two groups of people for recruitment as suitable provers, medical and non-medical. He stresses the advantages of the first group, commenting that physicians will know best the provings they have experienced personally.[8] But, in addition, he also gives detailed instructions for the procedure when physicians observe provings carried out by other people.[9] For both groups he requires high personal standards, stating that the chosen subjects should be trustworthy, intelligent, sensitive and unbiased.[10] His instructions then refer to the life-style of provers before and during the experiments and how their reports should be carefully recorded.

Many of the detailed instructions concern the diet of provers during the experiment. Hahnemann's requirements here are similar to his advice on the diet for people taking homoeopathic medicines therapeutically, namely simple, nourishing fresh food, as free as possible from medicinal herbs and stimulants.[11] In addition to the dietary demands, he requires that provers avoid excess exertion, mentally or physically, and pressure from urgent business. The translation by Dudgeon and Boericke of these instructions reads, "The person who is proving the medicine must during the whole experiment avoid all over-exertion of mind and body, all sorts of dissipation and disturbing passions; he should have no urgent business to distract his attention."[12] We may question how such directives could be strictly applied today, or indeed if they should be. It is arguable that provers testing medicines should do so when exposed to some degree of the stress factors likely also to influence the patients who will subsequently take the medicines therapeutically. This may have been Hahnemann's intention and that his instructions implied avoidance of excess rather than total prohibition. Hahnemann may simply have been recommending a lifestyle avoiding either deficiencies or excesses in such basic concerns as diet, rest, exercise, sex and business activities.

Having given instructions on the life-style of provers, Hahnemann turns his attention to the dose of the medicine to be taken and the recording of its effects. By the sixth edition of the *Organon* he was advising that provings should usually be conducted with potentized preparations, taken daily for a sufficient time for each individual to demonstrate the effects. The dosage strength and timing were therefore to be adjusted according to the individual prover's response, being sufficient to clarify the effects without provoking an excess reaction.[13] Again we see Hahnemann's respect for the individual reactions of people to medicinal stimuli. All the data were to be recorded, noting any symptoms produced, their intensity and their timing. Provers were also required to test medicines for changes of effect in differing situations, for instance indoors or outside, sitting still or exercising, eating or drinking.[14] Although, as we noted in an earlier chapter, Hahnemann did not himself use the term "modalities", these are implicit here. To help preserve accuracy from non-medical provers Hahnemann required that all the reports should be checked by physicians.[15]

It is evident from Hahnemann's writings that he saw these provings as important scientific studies to be conducted with precise care and reported in meticulous detail. Their primary aim was, and still is, the collection of data, as unbiased as possible by peculiarities of life-style or other activities of individual provers, and hopefully therefore suitable for application in therapy. All of this is important, but it is still only a superficial aspect of the gross data made available in provings. As Hahnemann reminds his readers many times, although such data are of basic importance they are not the whole or only intent of provings.

Hahnemann states that the collection of the data in provings has a deeper aim for the individual prover in training him to be a sharper observer of human function. Whilst provings are intended to be an assessment of the gross symptoms they evoke, they are also a challenge to us to observe, as closely as possible, the means through which such reactions occur. Looking for the effects produced in a proving, especially if we are doing it personally, can be like clarifying details of symptoms in the manner needed for an accurate assessment of a disease process. In both we may reflect sufficiently on what is happening, to observe details of physical effects as well as changes of emotions or thought patterns with which they correlate. Provings can be another aid towards rediscovering the continual interfunction between our thoughts, feelings and physical activities. In other words, they can heighten self-understanding.

Hahnemann summarizes his belief concerning these two aspects of the possible results from provings when he says, "Firstly, they bring home to him [the prover] . . . that what is medicinal in all medicines . . . lies in the disease conditions and changes in health which he has experienced in proving them. Secondly, such noteworthy observations on himself lead him to an understanding of his own sensations, the way he thinks and feels . . . something no physician can dispense with — they make him an observer."[16]

Hahnemann pursues the subtle implications of provings when he asserts that a spiritual essence contained within the medicinal agent is the active principle that interacts with similar dynamism within the organism of the prover. His suggestion is that this hidden component, which he terms the essence of the medicine, is particularly suited to interact with corresponding hidden energies within the recipient.[17] He termed the corresponding energies in the person taking medicine, "the vital force". Today we could describe them as psychological determinants. It is another aspect of the saying, let likes be treated by likes. If provings are pursued to this degree they can become a reminder to a prover of subtle energies operating in his own person. Hence Hahnemann's argument that self-provings can assist not only a better knowledge of medicinal effects, but also self-understanding that, quoting Greek philosophers, he terms "the essence of all true wisdom".[16]

Hahnemann's personal experiences of testing these subtle medicinal influences and their associated gross effects in the treatment of diseases led him progressively to formulate his views on primary and secondary reactions. As we noted in the previous chapter, he applied the term "primary reaction" to the initial disturbance of the vital force and associated symptoms produced in a human body by a medicine. The term "secondary reaction" was applied to the vital-force response, its attempt to rectify this change. A proving is therefore intended particularly to show the primary effect, the symptoms associated with the initial vital-force disturbance, and therefore the effect to be correlated with symptoms of a disease when applied therapeutically.[18]

Such a correspondence between the prior symptoms of a disease and the initial effect a remedy can provoke is not only the basis of homoeopathic prescribing, it is also the cause of the initial aggravation of symptoms sometimes seen when homoeopathic medicines are taken. Such an aggravation of symptoms shows that the primary action of the medicine matches particularly closely with the original disease and is therefore an accurate simillimum. Despite such reassurance most of us would rather avoid such an effect. We naturally dislike disease and prefer not to aggravate it. The possibility of an aggravation of symptoms, and I stress possibility because it appears only in a minority of patients, is so well known today that people having homoeopathic medicine for the first time often ask if it will worsen symptoms before it improves them. Homoeopathic practitioners often have to reassure patients new to homoeopathy that such aggravations or worsenings of symptoms are now only occasionally evident. In practice the intensification of the disease is usually unnoticed by the patient even though it is sufficient to provoke the healing, secondary action.

It appears from accounts of Hahnemann's early work that in the initial stages of his practice, when he used doses of medicines larger than those commonly used in his own later years and still prescribed today, that aggravations of symptoms fairly often preceded their improvement. This led Hahnemann to develop a technique of preparing progressively finer doses of the medicines required.

In practice, he found that these substantially decreased doses, or "potencies", as he termed them, for which homoeopathy has subsequently become famous to some, infamous to others, still produced the therapeutic effect required of the similia but were less likely first to produce an aggravation.[19] Hahnemann deduced that the appropriately reduced dose was able to arouse the vital force to counteract its own disturbed patterns and therefore correct the disease process, but was not enough to produce a tangible aggravation of the prior symptoms. Hence the reduced forms, or potencies, became regularly used in his practice of homoeopathic medicine.

Hahnemann's writings show that to him the size of the dose given was very important. He places progressive emphasis on finding the correct strength as well as correct form of a medicine for a particular patient. In his early writings, such as the first edition of the *Organon*, he refers to using the smallest dose of medicine required to assist healing but does not at that stage refer to potencies or potentization. These ideas develop subsequently, with prominence in his later works, particularly the sixth edition of the *Organon*.

REFERENCES

1. *Organon* 6th Edition   Paras 21, 25, 27, 105, 106
2. Ibid.   Paras 25a, 108, 120, 126
3. *Organon* 6th Edition   Para 270g trans. Künzli, Naudé and Pendleton
4. *Organon* 6th Edition   Para. 270 footnotes trans. Dudgeon and Boericke
5. *Organon* 6th Edition   Paras 119, 120, 143
6. Ibid.   Paras 116, 117
7. Ibid.   Para. 110
8. Ibid.   Para. 141
9. Ibid.   Paras 139–140
10. Ibid.   Paras 126, 141
11. Ibid.   Para. 125
12. *Organon* 6th Edition   Para. 126 trans. Dudgeon and Boericke
13. *Organon* 6th Edition   Paras 128, 129
14. Ibid.   Para. 133
15. Ibid.   Para. 139
16. *Organon* 6th Edition   Para. 141a trans. Künzli, Naudé and Pendleton
17. *Organon* 6th Edition   Paras 16, 269
18. Ibid.   Para. 114
19. Ibid.   Paras 159, 161

CHAPTER VIII

The Preparation of Homoeopathic Medicines

TO MANY PEOPLE homoeopathy is better known for its
use of very small doses of medicines than for the similia
principle implicit in its name and fundamental to its function. Even in medical meetings, where a correct use of the
term might be expected, it not infrequently happens that
"homoeopathy" is used to describe under-dosage with any
type of medication. Weak tea or coffee has sometimes been
called "homoeopathic". Although such a use of the term is
erroneous it is another indication of the spreading influence
of homoeopathy. Its language has crept into popular
vocabulary.

Clearly Hahnemann's training as a chemist proved useful
when he devised methods for preparing homoeopathic
medicines. He was able to develop ways of extracting them
from a range of sources as various as plants, shrubs, minerals
and animal products. Detailed lists of the sources of
medicines are found in his writings on materia medica. In
the *Organon*, as we noted in the previous chapter, he is more
concerned with their preparation and assessments of how
they achieve their effects than with their origins. However,
some references to the source materials occur when
Hahnemann gives instructions about the collection of specimens from which medicines are to be extracted. As well as
requiring that these should be as fresh as possible, or
carefully preserved if coming from abroad, he insists that
they should always be accurately named and that there are
advantages in using indigenous plants which are easier to
acquire.[1]

His aim was to develop a method that would release the
particularly active radical that he believed was an essential

component of the gross medicine whether animal, vegetable or mineral. He called the medicines produced "potencies" and the method of preparing them "potentization", or as it is sometimes termed "dynamization". This process was intended to release or unlock the essential nature of the medicinal agent and present it in a manner that could be applied therapeutically. It therefore included techniques intended to expose the powerful essential forms that Hahnemann believed were veiled by the ordinary gross presentation of the medicines.[2]

Hahnemann's copious writings show the gradual development of his ideas concerning potencies and his related instructions on how to prepare them. His early works, including the first edition of the *Organon*, refer only to using the smallest dose of medicine required to assist healing. Small doses were apparently advised to reduce side-effects or aggravations of symptoms. That is, they were intended to weaken the action of the medicine. Ideas concerning an enhancement of the effect through material reduction and succussion of medicines appear to have developed after Hahnemann observed the therapeutic responses to his prescriptions. It was a reversal of his previous deductions and led on to the use, in his later works, of the term "potency" to refer to the power forms that he believed were exposed in his medicines, and "potentization" for the method of their production.

He advised that for plants the sap should first be pressed out and mixed with alcohol, then left to stand and later decanted ready for further stages in the process. He varied the details according to the state of the plant. For dry plants he advised reducing them to a fine pulp prior to mixing with alcohol. He found that those with more mucilage required double the amount of alcohol needed for other plants. In addition he developed a method for drying powdered extracts of plants so that they could be stored for future use in preparing homoeopathic medicines.[1]

The process of potentization included grinding down the

crude form of the medicine and spreading it amongst milk sugar granules in a process termed "trituration". The product was then dissolved in a mixture of alcohol and distilled water and further prepared through a series of dilutions together with rhythmic shakings known as "succussion".

Hahnemann's directions for these processes are given in progressive detail. Trituration implied grinding one grain, by weight, of the gross form of the medicine with a pestle in a mortar containing 100 grains of powdered milk sugar. It was done in three stages with a third of the milk sugar used first, then another third added and then the final part. The aim was to spread the original grain as evenly as possible through the granules. Hahnemann's detailed instructions for this process include the timing for each stage. The completion of the three stages was to take one hour. The 1:100 ratio prepares the first centesimal or 1C triturate which can then be stored for further use later, or have one grain removed and treated in a similar manner with another 100 grains of milk sugar to prepare the 2C form. This again can either be stored or used immediately for further stages in the process.[3] Hahnemann found that at the 3C stage of trituration many substances, naturally insoluble in alcohol-water, have changed sufficiently to become soluble in this medium. This greatly facilitates the subsequent stages of potentization which can then be continued with the soluble form.

After trituration of previously insoluble substances, Hahnemann required that one grain of milk sugar into which the medicinal agent had been ground should be dissolved in 500 drops of alcohol ready for further serial dilutions and succussions. For the first stage in this liquid phase of the process one drop of this solution was further diluted in 100 drops of alcohol followed by the vigorous shaking of succussion. A drop of this solution in another 100 drops of diluent and again succussed gave the next stage, and so on.[4] For medicines naturally soluble in their original state Hahnemann advised using the liquid stages of potentization from the start.[5] Most of Hahnemann's work employed centesimal potencies, that is, dilutions and succussions on the 1:100 series at each stage. Later in this chapter we will refer to his use of other scales of potentization.

By the time Hahnemann was writing the sixth edition of the *Organon* he was mainly using 30C potencies, that is the 30th centesimal. This term implies that the serial dilution and succussion of one part of the medicated solution in 100 parts of diluent has been repeated 30 times. For each stage Hahnemann required fresh equipment and, for the succussions, 100 impacts on a firm surface such as that afforded by a leather-bound book. The product for each stage had to be labelled in its own vial. For long-term storage he advised moistening sugar globules with the medicated solution, allowing these to dry on filter paper, then storing the globules in labelled glass bottles protected from light. His instructions imply a remarkable level of industry and attention to detail.[6]

In the sixth edition of the *Organon* Hahnemann refers briefly to an extension of his ideas on the degrees and scales of potentization when he recommends preparing potencies from a solution of one part of the medicinal agent in 50,000 parts of diluent. He mentions this only briefly, but claims that such potencies achieved even better therapeutic effects than those previously prescribed.[7] Such comments occur only in this final edition of the *Organon*, written in the last decade of Hahnemann's life. This raises the question of whether they were more in the nature of theoretical deductions, and less tried in practice than his ideas of similia and their application with 30C potencies.

Hahnemann claims that trituration has an important effect in starting the progressive release of the essential form of the medicine from its relatively gross state. His writings indicate his understanding that all medicines, whether animal, vegetable or mineral, have a hidden, essential form capable of producing characteristic effects and that these can be released through the frictive processes of trituration and succussion.[8] One of the English translations refers to these processes as "unveiling" this essential form.[9] Hahnemann clearly regarded potentization as capable of enhancing the medicine's activity by releasing this highly active form or potency. At various times the process of preparation is referred to by terms subsequently translated as potentization, dynamization, transformation or spiritualization. All these terms imply changing the structure of the medicine to expose an active radical contained within it. Hahnemann compares this change of state to the development of magnetism by friction in an otherwise inert steel rod.

Whatever our assessment at this stage of Hahnemann's deductions concerning potentized medicines, their nature and how to prepare and use them, we can see that they pursue his two-fold ideals of attention to both gross and subtle aspects of any process, and of noting its own highly individual form of action. He sought to release the fundamental essence contained in the gross form of the particular medicine so that it could be used to stimulate the similarly hidden energies that govern our individual health or disease. He also frequently observes that each medicine has an effect characteristic to its type. He even calls it a law of nature. The previous chapter referred to the provings in which he sought to clarify such individual effects of medicines so that they could be matched with particular types of disease and used for treatment. In his instructions on the preparation of medicines he therefore insists on obtaining pure, accurately named products with the use of fresh glassware at each stage in the process. He was striving to obtain uncontaminated preparations of individual medicines, able to treat the dynamic causes of individual disease processes with which they correlated. This is the practical goal embodying his theoretical ideals.

The correspondence between the causes of diseases, and medicines able to treat them, applies both to the quality of the operant energies and the form of their effect. In other words, as Hahnemann deduces, finding the required similia involves matching both the quality of the energies determining the disease with those most effective in the medicine; and the form of symptoms seen in the disease with those that the medicine can produce in a healthy person.[10] Hence his emphasis on the importance of succussion to expose the hidden dynamism of medicines, and on the need always to match the individual picture presented in a disease process with carefully observed details of individual drug provings. His aim in therapy is to apply a medicinal stimulus correct in both its quality and form of effect for a specific disease process.

Hahnemann's application of these concepts in practice and the selection of the individual similia for an individual patient, will be the theme of the next chapter.

REFERENCES

1. *Organon* 6th Edition   Paras 266–268
2. Ibid.   Para. 269
3. Ibid.   Para. 270a
4. Ibid.   Para. 270
5. *Chronic Diseases*   Preface to 5th Volume. Hahnemann
6. *Organon* 6th Edition   Para. 270 and footnotes
7. Ibid.   Paras 270f,g
8. Ibid.   Paras 11a, 20, 269 and footnotes
9. *Organon* 6th Edition   Para. 11a trans. Dudgeon and Boericke
10. *Organon* 6th Edition   Paras 11a, 16, 148

CHAPTER IX

The Prescription of Homoeopathic Medicines

HAHNEMANN DESCRIBES THE selection of a homoeopathic medicine as an "arduous search" requiring "great circumspection and serious reflection".[1] The paragraph of the *Organon* that contains this comment also includes strong criticism of those practitioners who select a homoeopathic medicine from inadequate data, find it does not work, blame homoeopathy as deficient instead of themselves, and too quickly employ other treatment. He describes them as a "mongrel sect". Whilst such comments do not necessarily imply that Hahnemann always refused to advise non-homoeopathic treatment, they clearly show his contempt for a casual use of homoeopathy with a deficient response blamed on the process rather than its practitioner.

How, then, does Hahnemann proceed with his arduous search for a correct homoeopathic prescription? His writings show that he required a detailed as well as wide-ranging review of patients' diseases that could then be correlated with similarly detailed accounts of the pathogenic effects of medicines. That is, the symptoms they can induce in healthy people. His concern for appropriate attention to all aspects of the patients' symptoms is emphasized when he warns prescribers of the possible errors of being side-tracked by trivial complaints, on one hand, or too preoccupied with dominant features, on the other. Either way, the comprehensive and individual assessment required by Hahnemann would be impaired. An example of such errors, today, would be concentrating too much on a cosmetic change, such as a skin rash, and failing to notice an associated major disease, or being so preoccupied with the internal changes experienced by the patient, that the skin changes and their importance to the sufferer are ignored. To Hahnemann either of these would be an error falling short of the comprehensive review of disease processes that he required for precise homoeopathic prescribing.

Hahnemann's pursuit of these ideals has two aspects. The first points out the need to find a simillimum for the individual disease process at the moment it is presented. This is always important to Hahnemann's prescribing. The second aspect applies particularly in the treatment of chronic, long-standing disease. It draws attention to the role, in the present symptoms, of miasms, the lingering traces of old disease processes.

The search for a simillimum for a patient's disease involves taking a detailed review of the symptoms presented and their development, as already discussed earlier in this book. The detailed review Hahnemann required can then be correlated with the reports of provings or toxicology to advise an appropriate simillimum.

The other emphasis in prescribing concerns the use of anti-miasmatic agents. As we noted before, miasms are traces of long-standing disease patterns that may lie dormant in a person, but influence their vulnerability to harmful stimuli encountered later on, with these two factors then combining to produce obvious and often chronic disease symptoms. Effective therapy for diseases provoked in this way, Hahnemann argues, may therefore also require medicines particularly suited to treat this miasmic component.

Hahnemann gives a detailed discussion of chronic diseases in his book with that name. In the introduction entitled "Nature of Chronic Diseases", he advises making careful assessments of patients' symptoms going back long before the relatively recent changes reported, in order to assess a primitive disorder that he believed lingered and influenced the present disease state. An example would be including data about chicken-pox when someone's symptoms, whatever their present form, appear to start from such a problem. More complicated and controversial is Hahnemann's opinion that all long-standing disease develops from primitive medical disorders, particularly skin eruptions, experienced either in a person's own infancy or by his parents, with traces passed on.

Hahnemann pursues these theories, and their application in therapy, when he refers in the *Organon* to three particular groups of diseases. The first group he terms defective or local,[2] the second mental,[3] and the third intermittent diseases.[4] For each group his discussions have general applications as well as their particular emphasis. We will look at these more closely.

With some patients Hahnemann admits that a wide-ranging review of their symptoms is difficult. This may be because they have failed to notice changes in their health, or have convinced themselves that such effects are part of a normal cycle and therefore not worth reporting. He therefore advises that care should be exercised in history-taking, to watch out for such hazards. But in addition he admits that there are some diseases in which the effects are particularly localized and the symptoms relatively few.[5] When they produce mainly external changes he describes them as "local diseases". An example would be a skin rash with minimal evidence of an accompanying general reaction. Closely related to such localized forms of disease are those described by Hahnemann as "defective". He uses this term when symptoms are again few in number, but have an internal rather than external emphasis. An example would be a mood change considered notable enough to be termed a disease but without additional symptoms reported, or a headache difficult to locate and with few clear qualifying features.

Hahnemann keeps to his basic theory of disease when he recurrently asserts that even such local or defective diseases, despite their limited presentation, are superficial effects of inner hidden dynamic changes that must be taken into account for adequate therapy.[6] When he advises on the treatment for this group of diseases he therefore again insists that the assessment is as detailed as possible and includes data of long past disorders that may have left behind miasms that could contribute to the present picture. He then applies his two-fold approach of selecting both a simillimum for the recent symptoms, and an anti-miasmatic for lingering effects of old diseases.[7]

Hahnemann's discussions of local and defective diseases also contain some of his directives concerning how to take or apply the medicines selected. At first he argues against a combined use of medicines applied externally and taken internally. He deduces that the externally applied agent could lead to a deceptive disappearance of the superficial changes while leaving the deeper aspects of the disease process uncorrected and more difficult to detect.[8] These comments relate to the application of homoeopathic remedies. Hahnemann speaks even more strongly against the surface application of non-homoeopathic treatments, arguing that these not only prematurely remove the pointers to effective treatment, but cause the disease process to be driven back into the patient and increase its strength.[9] However, in the last paragraphs of the *Organon* he appears less resistant to applications of medicines in certain conditions. He admits that long-standing diseases may be helped by applying, locally, medicines that would also be effective when taken orally.[10]

These comments, and several statements by Hahnemann in the *Organon* paragraphs on local and defective diseases, raise issues highly relevant for homoeopathic prescribing today. This subject will be looked at more closely in the next chapter which refers to the interfunction of homoeopathy and other forms of therapy. But it is relevant also to introduce it here, as these discussions contain some particularly strong words from Hahnemann that may appear to condemn any combined use of homoeopathic remedies and other treatment. First we need to remember that Hahnemann was writing mainly in the early nineteenth century when other methods of therapy were often highly toxic as well as unpleasant. Second we may observe that he, too, at times allowed for other intervention that appeared necessary for urgent treatment. He cites the example of severe accidents needing prompt non-homoeopathic medical or surgical help.[11] Third, with many of the therapies available today, that appear safe as well as usefully effective, a strong case can be made for using an appropriate combined approach. The ideal of understanding and treating the causes of diseases need not necessarily exclude the use of appropriate palliative measures whilst people continue their attempts to rectify the hidden roots of the problems. Care is needed to help individuals clarify their own wishes in such choices.

The second of Hahnemann's three illustrative groups of diseases are those with an emphasis on mental symptoms. Here again his writings provoke the question of how his ideals are to be applied in the present day.

Hahnemann observed two main groups of mental illness. For one group he observed that physical symptoms preceded the psychological emphasis.[12] For the other group, that mental changes occurred without obvious physical effects coming first.[13] For an example of a mental disorder that follows obvious physical symptoms he refers to insanity developing after severe lung disease. It was a transition that at times appeared life-saving. As the symptoms shifted from a major physical emphasis, for instance severe respiratory difficulties, to psychological effects such as "melancholy or mania", the threat to life appeared to recede. This type of transition between physical and psychological symptoms is less often seen today than would have been likely in Hahnemann's lifetime. Modern methods of treatment frequently ease the effects of diseases reducing such manifestations. But the theory remains an interesting and important one, reminding us to look for all aspects of disease processes and still today to watch for signs, probably less sharp than in Hahnemann's era, of such a shifting emphasis during the course of a disease. All aspects, as he says many times, are relevant to the overall assessment.

Hahnemann deduced that mental symptoms preceded by

those with a physical emphasis indicated a more severe or deeper-rooted disease than those where psychological problems are dominant from the start. His description implies that the diseases he included in this more severe category are those that today would probably be called "psychoses". Although today obvious physical symptoms are not necessarily required as a prelude to diseases likely to be described as psychoses, the severity and type of disturbance arguably warrants their inclusion in Hahnemann's group of deeply rooted mental problems.

For their treatment he again refers to the need for careful assessment of organic and psychological effects and then advises treatment with an anti-psoric medicine as well as a simillimum. He suggests giving a simillimum prescription first and then, if needed for additional help later, adding an anti-miasmatic remedy.[14] He particularly refers to using anti-psoric, or occasionally anti-syphilitic medicines for such patients. His argument again is that although a simillimum may usefully reduce recent symptoms, if the disease relapses, a treatment taking more account of latent disease traits activated to produce the present disease, is likely to give longer relief.

That the prescription of medicine was not Hahnemann's only concern is shown by his emphasis on due attention to general care. He instructs that patients' attendants should always maintain a correct attitude to them. This, he advises, should be supportive, calm, accepting and without reproach. Such positive recommendations balance the negative aspects of his warnings against appeals to reason with severely disturbed patients.[15] He argues that they already sense their inability, for the time being, to change their behaviour by their own efforts, and that moral coercion therefore reminds them of their difficulties and aggravates their frustration.[16] These deductions again imply Hahnemann's careful observations of patients' behaviour. He noted that in those showing the mental disorders that he regards as particularly deep-rooted, their personal identity has been disturbed to such a degree that they are temporarily unable to direct their own thought processes and other responses, so that reasoning reminds them of their problems and aggravates their reactions to them.

He contrasts this type of mental illness with his second group. These are patients who today would probably be described as neurotic rather than psychotic. His description here implies a psychological disorder where the person's sense of identity holds although he experiences difficulties with his thought processes or emotions. An example would be a patient experiencing anxiety or depression who, despite the symptoms, retains his personal identity and his ability to reassess and modify his actions to some degree, especially if given appropriate help. Hence Hahnemann advises reasoning with him as well as prescribing an appropriate homoeopathic medicine.[17] Today a suitable form of psychotherapy might be recommended as well as a homoeopathic prescription.

Hahnemann's directives on the treatment of mental illness consistently imply, and at times firmly state, his respect for the individual authority of each person. He accepts that, although the individual capacity for self-direction may be impeded during mental illness, it is not removed and is still to be respected.[18]

Hahnemann's theories concerning these two groups of mental diseases are easier to follow if we recall that our bodies are energy fields and their diseases due to rearrangements of these energetic patterns. Psychosis may be regarded as a disease in which the disturbed patterns are of such strength that the individual cannot at that moment apply his own understanding and will power sufficiently to correct the imbalance. The inertia of the disease process at that stage overcomes an individual's capacity to control it. Hence additional help is required to ease the disturbance and enable the patient to regain his own control. In contrast to this, with neurosis, the degree of disturbance is enough to be a problem and lead to symptoms, but at that stage does not totally overrule the individual's capacity for conscious control. The disruption is not so severe. Homoeopathic medicines and appropriate forms of psychotherapy can help individuals who experience this type of disorder to work through their difficulties towards increased personal health.

The third group of disorders given particular attention by Hahnemann were called intermittent diseases. Here he was concerned particularly with intermittent episodes of fever, often due to malaria, common in his day. However, since Hahnemann recorded his views, the use of a range of preventative and therapeutic measures developed for malaria has significantly altered its impact. It may therefore be suggested that his ideas on this subject are irrelevant today. The discussion of Hahnemann's theories on intermittent diseases need not however, be restricted to malaria. The insights that he developed in relation to that particular problem arguably also have a general application for other regularly relapsing disorders. Recurring conditions for which homoeopathic treatment is often sought today include such common problems as hay fever, dysmenorrhoeoa (period pains) and migraine. These, and many other common diseases, tend to recur on a regular basis. It may therefore be reasoned that Hahnemann's theories on the treatment of regularly relapsing diseases are in many ways applicable to such present day problems.

Hahnemann distinguished two groups of such disorders. In the first, relative health alternates with episodes of disease. In the second, there is an alternation between two particular forms of disease.[19] An example of the first group would be a person experiencing hay fever in the usual season but feeling well for the rest of the year. The second group is exemplified by the people who alternate between asthma and eczema. As one problem eases the other takes over.

The usual expectation of patients today is that symptoms will be treated as they arise. For intermittently relapsing diseases, however, Hahnemann advises a different regime. He recommends that it may be appropriate to prescribe a suitable remedy as the attack subsides.[20] He argues that at this stage the body may be freer from the more severe effects of the paroxysm and therefore better able to respond effectively with a thorough correction of the disturbance so that not only are the vestiges of the present episode cleared, but subsequent recurrence is less likely. If, however, a relapse still occurs later on, he advises that even if the similar form of medicine is indicated, its potency can be slightly enhanced by further succussion.[21] For the choice of remedy he advises that this should correlate with as many features as possible of the whole picture. This implies taking into account all the features of the various phases when prescribing for any particular stage of the disease.[22] It is a development of his attention to all aspects of recent disease symptoms when prescribing a simillimum.

In addition to this, Hahnemann again argues the value of an anti-miasmatic agent. He reasons that relapse of the disease process after a simillimum has been prescribed, and aggravating environmental factors removed, may indicate a persisting miasmic disorder for which a further homoeopathic remedy is required.[23]

For all of these three groups of diseases referred to particularly by Hahnemann in his illustrations of the application of homoeopathic medicines, we see his continual insistence on prescribing for a careful and highly detailed review of present symptoms, and applying similar care to the selection of remedies for persisting traits of old diseases, as miasms may be described. In Hahnemann's day the pursuit of such ideals must have implied a great deal of memorizing and checking the data from provings. Since then the selection of medicines has been helped by the availability of "repertories". These are reference books that resemble dictionaries; they list particular symptoms and their modalities for each part of the body. They are very useful aids to cross-checking the remedies suitable for each individual feature of a disease process and eventually choosing one that seems to apply for most of them. Today this process is made even easier with the aid of computerized repertories. This is not saying that computers can prescribe a homoeopathic remedy. They are merely aids to the assessment which still rests between patients and therapists as together they evaluate and assess symptoms for the selection of a suitable simillimum.

In his writings on prescribing for local, mental and intermittent diseases Hahnemann refers several times to particular pointers to watch for when selecting second or subsequent prescriptions. He expands these ideas in subsequent paragraphs of the *Organon* when he considers the principles that generally relate to the prescribing of homoeopathic medicines.

Of primary importance is Hahnemann's insistence on a reappraisal of the prescribing needs before any repeat prescription is selected. The follow-up consultation allows a review of changes in old symptoms, noting of any new ones that have developed and, often important, revision of previous reports. The span and depth of the assessment for homoeopathic prescribing is such that people often return on their second or subsequent visit with reports of symptoms they forgot to mention or described inadequately last time.

Hahnemann distinguishes several types of response to treatment often still seen today, and advises on the associated modifications of the prescriptions.[24] For a prompt and steadily progressing improvement of the symptoms he advises against repetition of the prescription. This is more likely with acute diseases. For symptoms of chronic diseases improvement usually takes longer. When symptoms improve only slowly, Hahnemann recommends repeating the medicine but with slight variations in its potency achieved by additional succussions between doses. When there is no improvement at all in the previously reported symptoms, also perhaps a slight sign of a proving associated with the medicine given, Hahnemann advises a complete reassessment and selection of a new prescription. In some diseases, particularly those presenting with localized effects, he observes that after treatment is started new symptoms sometimes arise that are part of the original disorder and have been aroused through the first prescription. He regards this development as part of the process required for healing, implying that it is releasing the disease that can then be corrected as the additional symptoms enable the selection of an even more suitable homoeopathic medicine.[25]

A possible reaction discussed several times by Hahnemann is a brief worsening of initial symptoms, termed an aggravation. As we discussed in a previous chapter, Hahnemann observed this effect early in his homoeopathic practice but reduced its occurrence through developing the process of potentization and prescribing infrequent doses of the minute medicinal stimuli that he called potencies. In the *Organon* he therefore observes that aggravations, though unlikely to be severe, may arise if a homoeopathic prescription is given in a form that is not appropriately potentized or is repeated too soon for a particular individual.[26] If they occur he regards them as a sign of an accurate prescription that will be followed by a useful improvement of symptoms [27] and for their treatment simply advises stopping the prescription.[28] We need to be careful in assessing apparent aggravations of symptoms. True exacerbations of previous disease processes, that can be expected to improve steadily and clear if treatment is stopped, need to be distinguished from new symptoms of a continuing disease which has not responded to treatment and requires reassessment for a different prescription.

Closely related to these observations on second or subsequent prescriptions are Hahnemann's comments on the factors that can hinder a therapeutic response. Having observed that patients sometimes appear to be no better even though they have had a medicine that seems clearly indicated for their needs, he deduces that impedances or "obstacles to cure" may be getting in the way.[29] Amongst the impedances he includes many dietary ingredients that he considered unhelpful, emotional trauma, too much or too little exercise or sleep, certain forms of clothing and poor housing. These are practical points sometimes interpreted by Hahnemann's readers today as implying that patients having homoeopathic treatment should have no coffee or tea and avoid strong toothpaste. Hahnemann's comments on diet for patients are similar to the advice he has given to provers. Much of it can be summarized as an avoidance of obvious stimulants and a preference for fresh, simple foods. The importance of a correct diet appropriate to personal needs and tolerances is increasingly acknowledged today. Since dietary advice is often sought in conjunction with homoeopathic treatment, we will look at it in more detail in the next chapter.

After the form of a medicine has been decided on, and obstacles to cure avoided as far as possible, we still need to select the potency with which to begin treatment and to decide on how frequently to give it. Hahnemann's attention to the individuality of every patient again shows itself when he advises adjusting the potency prescribed according to particular responses. His aim was to use the smallest medical stimulus that would provoke the appropriate vital force response for that individual. A potency too high or too low for the individual could, he argued, produce an unwanted aggravation of symptoms prior to an improvement, particularly when treating chronic disease. He therefore advised careful monitoring to check the patient's response, and adjustment of the prescription as required.

It is clear from his writings that Hahnemann did not regard the medicinal stimulus as the only one required for effective treatment. His writings also contain advice on other therapeutic measures some of which we have referred to briefly earlier in this chapter. Examples included advice on diets, rest, exercise and housing conditions. In addition he specifically recommends certain other forms of therapy that he regarded as useful additions to homoeopathic treatment. The question of which therapies can be usefully combined with homoeopathy is often asked. It is as important today as it was for Hahnemann.

REFERENCES

1. *Organon* 6th Edition   Para. 148a trans. Künzli, Naudé and Pendleton
2. *Organon* 6th Edition   Paras 172–203
3. Ibid.   Paras 214–230
4. Ibid.   Paras 231–244
5. Ibid.   Paras 173–175
6. Ibid.   Paras 189, 190, 201
7. Ibid.   Paras 195, 201–206
8. Ibid.   Paras 196–197
9. Ibid.   Para. 202
10. Ibid.   Para. 285
11. Ibid.   Paras 67a, 186
12. Ibid.   Paras 215–220
13. Ibid.   Paras 225–226
14. Ibid.   Paras 217–223
15. Ibid.   Paras 228–229
16. Ibid.   Paras 224, 224a
17. Ibid.   Para. 226
18. Ibid.   Para. 229
19. Ibid.   Paras 231, 232
20. Ibid.   Para. 236
21. Ibid.   Para. 238
22. Ibid.   Para. 235
23. Ibid.   Paras 240–243
24. Ibid.   Paras 246–250
25. Ibid.   Paras 179–182
26. Ibid.   Para. 160
27. Ibid.   Para. 158
28. Ibid.   Para. 281
29. Ibid.   Paras 3, 255, 259, 260

CHAPTER X

The Interfunction of Homoeopathy with other Therapies

IN ORDER TO make a fair appraisal of Hahnemann's views
on this important subject we need first to remind ourselves of
the time in which he was writing. Hahnemann was working
on the sixth edition of the *Organon* shortly before his death in
1843. His particular recommendations in that book therefore concern the therapies available then. However, this
need not necessarily restrict our review to the situation that
applied in the nineteenth century. Hahnemann's specific
comments on a combined application of homoeopathy and
some of the medical practices available in his day contain
points of a general validity still applicable today.

On first reading the *Organon*, or other writings by
Hahnemann, it is very easy to get the impression that he was
absolutely opposed to any prescription of non-homoeopathic
medicines. He frequently and firmly denounces the problems that he believed arose from their use. However, on
closer reading we will find occasional admissions that they
have some therapeutic validity. An example occurs in his
acknowledgement that an emergency such as drowning may
require medicines of a non-homoeopathic form since a
simillimum in this case would not be sufficiently fast acting.[1]
Although we referred, in the previous chapter, to the
principles involved here, they are of such importance to the
practice of homoeopathy today that we will again pursue
them.

Another acknowledgement by Hahnemann that he had
not discovered homoeopathic medicines appropriate for all
forms of disease, occurs in his discussions of provings. Here
he admits that a vast range of provings would be needed to

find medicines likely to help, even partially, all forms of disease and this implies his admission that this goal was not realized in his time.[2] The situation is similar today. We do not know how to treat by homoeopathy all the disease states we see. Although many forms of acute and chronic diseases can be helped by homoeopathic medicines there are others which, at this stage in our knowledge, we cannot treat adequately in this way. Obviously, increasing our knowledge and understanding of homoeopathy will enable us to use it more extensively. But most homoeopathic prescribers readily admit that additional forms of therapy, including other medicines, are also required at times. This is why many of us welcome the use of the term "complementary" to describe homoeopathy. The implications of this word are far more relevant today than the idea of choosing homoeopathy *or* other therapy, as was suggested in the past when it was described as an "alternative medicine". Naturally homoeopathic practitioners prefer to use homoeopathic prescriptions as far as possible. But this need not prevent an appropriate use of other forms of medicine when they are required in conjunction with homoeopathy. Many examples could be given of homoeopathic medicines used in conjunction with non-homoeopathic forms of treatment, resulting in clear reports of benefits to patients with diseases as various as arthritis, colitis, eczema and anxiety states. For some patients with such problems homoeopathic medicines may be the only prescription required, but for others a combined approach has often been useful.

Hahnemann's attitude to surgery may at first also appear to be totally negative. Throughout his writings he recurrently asserts his view that all diseases, even those with an obvious local physical effect such as a lump in the wrong place, have a dynamic cause affecting the person as a whole, and that a homoeopathic simillimum is the ideal therapy. However, such an ideal does not prevent him from admitting that in certain circumstances surgical intervention is likely also to be required. He cites examples such as fractures, cut arteries, and penetrating wounds, calling them "the proper domain of surgery". Admittedly, such examples all refer to treatment of severe accidental injury. But a translation of the paragraph that allows for surgery in these cases, also refers to its relevance for "opening a body cavity to remove a substance causing trouble or to drain extravasated or collected fluids".[3] Such comments may be interpreted as an acceptance by Hahnemann of surgical intervention for problems arising from natural diseases as well as for effects of trauma. He adds a reminder that an appropriate homoeopathic medicine given concurrently can also offer effective help.

In assessing such comments today we need to recall that the surgery of Hahnemann's day was very different from the operative and anaesthetic techniques now available. It is hardly surprising that Hahnemann resisted many of the practices pursued in his time and therefore often appeared to be against the use of surgery. That even in his day he accepted the need for surgery for major trauma, and perhaps also for other causes of major physical difficulties, arguably implies that he would be even less opposed to an appropriate use of the far safer surgical procedures available now. His reminder that a homoeopathic prescription may be given concurrently is often acted on today. Whilst surgery is accepted for gross physical effects of disease, a homoeopathic prescription can at times also aid the recovery from the original pathology and the surgical intervention.

Hahnemann's continuing attention to the various aspects of health and disease shows itself again in his comments on the adjuvants to homoeopathic therapy. The previous chapter referred to his views on the treatment of mental diseases and his comments about aspects of care that today would be described as psychotherapeutic. We also noted his concern for due attention to physical needs such as appropriate housing, clothing, exercise and diets. Questions are often asked, nowadays, concerning dietary measures that can assist homoeopathic treatment. It is therefore appropriate to consider these questions again, and in more detail.

In general today there is much more concern about appropriate diets, as well as a growing awareness that some individuals react strongly to certain foods. Hahnemann expressed his opinions about diet long before its importance became a more accepted concern. His comments were strongly stated, often in a manner that sounds very restrictive. For instance, he advises that, especially for patients with chronic diseases, the diet should exclude a long list of items, amongst them coffee, china tea, herbal teas, certain beers, cordials, spiced chocolate, coffee and vanilla ice-cream, sprouting and medicinal vegetables, parsley, celery and onion, various meats and old cheese. After this list he comments that some of his "imitators unnecessarily make the patient's regimen even harder and forbid many more rather unimportant things".[4] It is a long list, too long for some of Hahnemann's critics. But whatever we decide for ourselves about Hahnemann's detailed recommendations on diet, surely his general insistence on having food that was as fresh and nourishing as possible, and not too stimulating or too much in quantity for the individual, was reasonable both for his day and for now? Again the emphasis on individual needs is evident. He allows that, especially in acute disease, it may be more helpful for a patient to eat what he feels he needs, within moderation.[5] In this situation Hahnemann asserts that the correct homoeopathic medicine can co-operate with the general contentment of the patient to assist healing. Today a correct diet for individual needs is clearly important. It is comparable to finding appropriate fuel for a car. An appropriate diet is important for patients with any form of disease, but it also needs to be acceptable to those concerned. Some of the regimes advocated today are at least as harsh as those advised by Hahnemann. Obviously, if there is clear benefit, patients and their families willingly accept difficult dietary measures. But care is needed in advising diets for general application. They are another area where individual assessment is required.

Other therapies discussed by Hahnemann, for possible use in his day as additional aids to healing, included mesmerism, animal magnetism, massage and bath therapy.[6] These four examples are no longer practised today as they were in the nineteenth century, but their contemporary replacements might be said to include hypnosis, therapeutic massage and hydrotherapy. Other techniques that are widely used today in conjunction with homoeopathy and, some practitioners would argue, share Hahnemann's ideal of appropriately stimulating the vital force to assist healing, include acupuncture and psychotherapy.

Today many forms of treatment are offered together with homoeopathy in the name of complementary medicine. The range includes not only such techniques as acupuncture, psychotherapy, hypnosis and dietary measures, but also lesser known techniques such as aroma therapy and iridology. It is often assumed that these are all close allies of homoeopathy, pursue similar ideals such as "natural" health care, and work well together. Caution is needed before such claims are accepted. Hahnemann's ideals concerning therapy posited that it would not only relieve symptoms of disease, but also help patients gain more understanding about themselves. He saw disease as a process that, if adequately assessed by both patient and therapist, can usefully increase human self-understanding. With some of the forms of therapy presented today there is more emphasis on physical needs and relaxation, and less on the gaining of insight. When that happens it may be argued that the treatment is not pursuing all the ideals encouraged by Hahnemann. For him therapy was only thoroughly effective if it included an intelligent research into the determinants of particular disease symptoms and did not merely focus on their anticipated removal. Although many forms of complementary medicine practiced today share this Hahnemann ideal, it cannot be said for all of them. Hence the need for caution before we assume that all such methods of treatment support Hahnemann's therapeutic goals.

Hahnemann's attention to diet, exercise, sleep, appropriate surgery and other clearly indicated and correctly applied medicines shows his concern for the physical aspects of health care. His corresponding attention to the more subtle factors is shown in his frequent references to emotional, ideological or spiritual determinants of health, disease and therapy. His writings imply that, as his work continued, he became increasingly aware of subtle causes of diseases and their role in therapeutic responses. Particular evidence of this trend occurs in his increasing references in his later years to an aspect of consciousness termed by him "Geistartigen Wesen", and subsequently translated into the English terms "spiritual" or "conceptual essences".

In several previous chapters of this study there have been references to these terms and Hahnemann's apparent attempts to indicate by their use an initiative or causal quality of consciousness. Arguably they are of such importance to the understanding developed by Hahnemann of the processes involved in homoeopathic medicine, and in other forms of therapy, that they warrant further review.

REFERENCES

1. *Organon* 6th Edition   Para. 67a
2. Ibid.   Para. 145
3. *Organon* 6th Edition   Para. 186 trans. Künzli, Naudé and Pendleton
4. Ibid.   Para. 260a
5. *Organon* 6th Edition   Para. 263
6. Ibid.   Paras 286–291

CHAPTER XI

Hahnemann's Theory of Conceptual Essences

HAHNEMANN'S USE OF German terms such as "Geistartigen Wesen", subsequently translated "conceptual" or "spiritual essences", occurs infrequently and only in his later writings.[1] Arguably such phrases express a profound insight gradually developed throughout his many years of research into the dynamics of health, disease and homoeopathic therapy. His writings reveal his constant determination to seek a fuller understanding of the hidden causes of visible physical effects. The works of his last decade, particularly the sixth edition of the *Organon*, express his mature insights, evolved through a long commitment to detailed and searching enquiry.

Before pursuing in detail the implications of conceptual-essence theories it is necessary to restate the basic awareness that *all* forms that exist are energy. Philosophers have said so for centuries, scientists are beginning to agree with them. A fundamental implication of the discovery that all matter is composed of power, is that there are, in fact, no static material forms. All the appearances of apparently static formal structures are due to particular patterns of movement. A simple illustration occurs when spinning a bicycle wheel. If it spins fast enough and maintains that pattern of movement, it looks and behaves as if it has solid form. A marble thrown against it is blocked and thrown off. The movement has produced both the appearance and activity of a substantial barrier.

A similar principle applies to all apparently material forms: they are patterns of energy. Particular motion patterns, or forms of energy, create the individual appearances of everything that exists. The world as a whole, its inhabitants, and anything they presume to make, are all dynamic, they are movements of energy. Our individual bodies, everything in our environment, anything existential we can name: all are dynamic structures.

Applied to our physical bodies this means that all their features, external and internal, are dynamic. Our external appearance, the shape of our bodies and their internal structures usually appear consistent from one day to the next because of repeated similar forms in their energy patterns. But in every moment this apparent continuity of form is composed of a dynamic flux.

There is no non-energy form in our bodies or in their environment.

Such an understanding of the form or shape of our bodies applies similarly to their function, the work they accomplish. This too is always an expression of the energy comprising them. Western minds in general have often found it easier to think of material rather than dynamic forms. It is easy to slip into dualistic or separatist-type thinking by assuming that function implies doing something with a "solid" form. Walking can be thought of as the function that might be shown when the decision to move is applied to an apparently static pair of legs. But this type of thought would be an erroneous dualism, or twoness, if it implied the idea that legs are only functional when applied in walking or some other defined movement. That is not the correct implication of the awareness that all forms are continually dynamic and functional. The fact that they exist implies that their constituent forces are moving constructively in every moment. Their existence is itself a function. Its expression is varied from moment to moment when, for instance, the legs are moved for walking after resting for a time. But function is never absent.

All the structures in our bodies, and any other form in their environment, are actually dynamic in every moment of their existence. Their form is how they appear at any moment, their function is the work they perform at the same time. These two aspects always go together. There is no possibility of a non-functional form, or a formless function.

An idea is another type of dynamic form and function. This time it is a mental process. Ideas are mental forms and they too are particular patterns of activity. Each idea conceived in our minds is due to energy operating in that manner, and has formal and functional aspects. Whether the thoughts are concerned with human understanding or house repairs, they are mental energies operating to produce the relevant images and having their own inherent functions.

The effects of thoughts can easily be forgotten, even though they are continually shown in our ordinary daily lives. When happy, relaxing thoughts occupy our minds we are more likely to experience and convey a similarly happy and relaxed mood in our physical behaviour. Conversely, if negative thoughts such as those of anger or resentment predominate, our physical characteristics will change accordingly. The expression may be masked, particularly in a person trained not to be emotionally demonstrative. But even here there will be a change observable to the person experiencing it, if he will acknowledge it to himself, as well as some subtle outward hint detectable to a trained eye.

The contrasting effects of positive pleasurable thoughts, as opposed to negative disturbing ones, have now been realized to such a degree that they have been applied therapeutically. Various psychotherapies include techniques intended to help people consciously apply pleasant images and thoughts to aid body relaxation. They have been used in conjunction with other forms of therapy by people with a wide range of medical problems, as various for instance as hypertension, cancer and phobic anxiety. The process usually involves a combined use of techniques to aid physical relaxation, and conscious imaging of pleasant relaxing activities, such as country walks, reading a good book or any other appropriate recreational pursuit.

It may be argued that Hahnemann anticipated such therapy long before its present application.[2] We noted in a previous chapter his emphasis in the *Organon* on the role of positive imagery in contributing to health or disease.

With the advances of modern science aiding us it is easier today than it would have been in the time of Hahnemann to assess the processes involved in such therapeutic techniques. The insight that all forms, whether mental constructs or physical organs, are energy patterns with their own essential functions, makes it easier to understand the continual interaction between thoughts, and similarly between dynamic gross bodies and thoughts. The old supposition that intangible thoughts merely *possibly* influence our material bodies is now demonstrably erroneous. Instead, the continual interaction of our thought life and physical activity is better compared to various streams of water mingling to produce a unified current.

Studies from medical practice further complement this understanding. For many years biology students have been taught the association between adrenalin output and fear. It has been termed the "fright and flight reaction". We know it in our own bodies. If we misjudge crossing a road and nearly have an accident, we feel fear, or even perhaps a panic reaction. The quickened pulse, skin cooling and sweating are today known to be associated with a surge of adrenalin provoked through extra activity of the autonomic nervous system and the adrenal glands. We know too that similar reactions can be provoked by thoughts or images. A clear example is the pre-flight anxiety of people phobic of flying. Their reactions, mentally and physically, to the idea of an impending flight, sometimes show clearly and strongly several days in advance of the actual take-off, especially in these days when aircraft are often a target for terrorism.

Other illustrations of such substantial effects of thoughts and emotions have come from studies of people who have experienced bereavement. Careful follow-up has demonstrated changes in white blood cells associated with bereavement reactions. Probably we all know from our personal experience that reactions such as grief, loneliness or at times anger after a major loss, change our body muscle tone. Often at such times people also experience increased physical tiredness, muscle tension or general lethargy. Such states sharply contrast with the tone of muscles etc. when things appear to be going well and there is a natural enthusiasm to get on with activities.

These experiences illustrate what may be called the "chemistry" of thoughts. They show that chemical or other physical effects are correlative with mental activity. Such effects are some of the functions of mental images referred to earlier in this chapter and they clearly illustrate the continuous influence of our thought processes on our physical activity and health.

They also illustrate the specific nature of the function of any given form. They show that the effect, or productive function, of each thought is integral and characteristic to its form. Not only do form and function always go together, but each form has a *specific* function, and each function a *specific* form. These are essential features of any concept and of any other structure including apparently "material" substance. They imply that for every activity man performs, whether it is mental or physical in emphasis, there will inevitably be a particular substantial effect.

Hahnemann frequently refers to such individual effects of particular forms of activity. He speaks of them in relation to the individual expressions of particular infections or other diseases when he reminds us to note that a patient has "a *kind* of St Vitus Dance" and not to assume that every person with a disorder so named has identical problems.[3] It is implicit in all his discussions on case-taking; he again refers to it frequently when he considers provings and the need to investigate the individual effects that each medicine can produce in relatively healthy people. In this part of his discussion he goes so far as to describe the occurrence of specific effects for each medicine as a "law of nature".[4]

Before we consider the implications of these insights in relation to Hahnemann's use of the term "conceptual essence" and its relevance to homoeopathic therapy, we need to note a third aspect of any activity, additional to the formal and functional qualities already observed. This is its cause. Again it is an aspect to which Hahnemann refers frequently in his writings. Many times in the previous chapters we have noted his attempts to understand the causes of human health and disease. The awareness of formal and functional aspects of any activity, itself implies that they have a cause. It is a triad of form, function and cause to which many philosophers and similar thinkers have referred. If our understanding of any process is to be thorough, this aspect clearly needs due attention. To neglect it would be like trying to understand the working of an electric light bulb without considering its power-source and switch.

References to conceptual or spiritual essences clearly refer to such causal aspects of reality. When the German term used by Hahnemann is translated "spiritual essence", the reference to causality is particularly evident. In philosophy the term spirit implies initiation. It is used similarly by religious thinkers in attempts to refer to an awareness of an original cause. In Wyld's *Universal English Dictionary* the term spirit is said to derive from a Latin term meaning "breath of life". Its etymology, philosophic and religious applications all therefore refer to an original living cause of the form and function shown. A similar implication can be seen in the term "essence". As is often said, nothing happens without a cause. The activity it denotes is vital, or essential, to the construct.

We may therefore deduce that in applying the term translated conceptual or spiritual essence, Hahnemann is referring to the cause, as well as the formal and functional aspects of the activities he studied.

The sixth edition of the *Organon* contains several particularly clear references to this cause. Hahnemann writes of observing events in the world as a whole, such as the movements of the moon and tides, and comments that it is not possible to detect a sequence of cause and effect. He describes it as a dynamic influence with no mechanical or material delay. Or, putting it another way, that the cosmic rhythm causing such events has an immediate effect so that no delay is detected between the causal impulse and the observed planetary motion and tidal response. He therefore implies that the initiative and compliance are not separated, and the volitional intent is integral to the responsive form.[5]

He then deduces that the contagious effect of an infectious disease, like measles, is also due to such a dynamic influence. He deduces that the invisible contagious force interacts with the similarly unseen causal consciousness in a human being to produce its characteristic physical effect. Here again, he implies that the compliance of the recipient is immediate because it is its own inherent will that is activated to provoke the response. It is therefore another example of a non-separation of the will and the responsive form.

In such discussions Hahnemann's basic insight is that the essential cause of change is the inherent will of the form itself. This may be aroused, when for instance the measles infection is encountered, but it is the subtle processes of the will of the recipient, in response to the stimulus received at a similarly dynamic level, that provoke the overt physical change. Again he applies the term "vital force", the concept widely used in his day in an attempt to refer to the unseen factors of life operating within our physical bodies. His intention here appears to be to compare the interaction between the sea and the cosmic determinative impulses, to that occurring between the visible processes of the human body, its own inherent and unseen will and the infectious stimulus to which it responds. In other words, he appears to be emphasizing by example the role of the will of the recipient to order its own form-function aspects in response to the similarly dynamic disease-provoking stimulus.

In the next stage of his argument he deduces that the medicinal effects of natural substances similarly occur when their spiritual or initiative aspects interact with the corresponding modality in a living body. He says, "Natural substances that have been found to be medicinal are so only by virtue of their power (specific to each one of them) to modify the human organism through a dynamic, spirit-like effect ... upon the spirit-like vital principle that governs life."[6] In other words, he is again deducing that a causal impulse operates within the form-function structure of the medicine and that this is accepted by the corresponding modality or will in the person who receives it, to produce the physical effects.

Hahnemann therefore appears to deduce that the physical effects of gross medicines are determined primarily by unseen causal aspects operating in the medicinal stimulus and the person who receives it. Applied in day-to-day experiences this would mean that an antacid for indigestion is effective, not only when irritant chemicals are moderated, but also and primarily, because of an unseen intent in the person who receives it. Perhaps this deduction relates to the apparent failure of some medicines to act even though they appear clearly indicated for the individual patient.

In all of these examples Hahnemann is referring back to the non-separation of cause and effect he has observed in the oceanic tides. The cause of the change seen is actually in the form responding. Even when the sea responds to a cosmic impulse, and the human body to infection or medicine, the essential cause of the effect is within the recipient-responding form. He implies that the will or control that provokes the change in the sea, or in human form, is integral to it and in immediate rapport with the compliant substance. It is the will of the form-function; and the form-function of the will. Hence there is no separation between cause and effect.

Hahnemann's references to conceptual essences therefore have increasingly profound implications. They refer to the dynamic nature of all constructs, mental or physical, their unique formal-functional aspects, and imply that the cause of the form-function is within itself. Pursuing the implications of such insight leads to some challenging concepts concerning our health and day-to-day function, as well as our responses to disease stimuli.

The individuality of every form-function complex implies the need to find for our own bodies those structures that are assimilable, remembering too that this applies to mental and apparently physical energy input. Just as assimilable energy intake, including homoeopathic similia, will enhance health, the unassimilable forms, particularly if they are retained, will impair it. This is readily observed for food that does not suit an individual. It is equally valid for ideas and other subtle stimuli.

These concepts also relate to the mode of action of homoeopathic medicines. They imply the capacity of a correct homoeopathic stimulus, naturally corresponding to the subtle processes of the recipient, to assist a reintegration of personal energies. In other words, the medicines can co-operate with the will of the recipient to re-order his or her own being.

Hahnemann's insights concerning causal aspects of all form-function units are not easily pursued, but are profoundly important. Related concepts of causal factors within human beings imply for us a capacity for true self-determination. This is a particularly challenging concept and will be explored further in the final chapter of this study.

REFERENCES

1. *Organon* 6th Edition   Paras
   11, 270
2. Ibid.   Para. 17a
3. Ibid.   Para. 81b
4. Ibid.   Para. 111
5. Ibid.   Paras 11, 11a
6. *Organon* 6th Edition   Para.
   11a trans. Künzli, Naudé and
   Pendleton

CHAPTER XII

The Necessity for Self-Understanding

IN GENERAL PRACTICE and hospital out-patient clinics today it is often apparent that many people prefer not to question their own basic anatomy and physiology. When the discussion appears likely to turn to such topics, often people will readily admit that they prefer not to know, and they will change the subject or get ready to leave, through fear. They see no need to try to understand their own constitution, preferring instead to leave such matters to trained medical advisers who they hope they will seldom need to consult. An example of this was shown by a patient giving her medical history who stated that she had had abdominal surgery but had no idea of what had been done. She said she "preferred not to know".

There is probably an even greater lack of questioning of our ideas and emotions, why we hold them and the effect they can have on our activities. It is all too easy to allow remembered likes or dislikes as well as ideas retained from many years ago, to prejudice decisions made today. Examples range from adults refusing to read Shakespeare because of memories of O-level examinations, to children refusing green vegetables because of memories of school meals. Such habits are frequently ignored and allowed to run unquestioned.

This attitude is a far cry from the ideal stated by Hahnemann and many other thinkers, including the Delphic Oracle, whose aim, as we noted in chapter I, was "know thyself". Hahnemann's concern with Self-understanding is implicit throughout the *Organon* as well as being stated openly when, for instance, he describes it as the "essence of all true wisdom".[1]

Confronted by these two contrasting attitudes, with searchers for insight opposed by those who are unconcerned, we may ask, why pursue *Self*-understanding? Why not hope all goes well, ask questions and seek help only if we run into obvious problems, and the rest of the time do whatever we enjoy? Hahnemann's writings imply two strong arguments against such an attitude, and for the pursuit of Self-knowledge and direction. One is the negative aspect, that lack of such understanding makes us more vulnerable to undetected problems. The other is more positive, that increased awareness of our individual possibilities places us in a better position to use and enjoy them.

The heightened vulnerability that correlates with a lack of self-knowledge is easily observed. It is comparable to not understanding a car we drive and suffering the consequences miles from anywhere on a cold, wet night. A few people become very attached to their cars, spend a lot of time, effort and money trying to understand and improve them and react strongly if they break down. Our bodies are our cars and a deficiency of understanding here can involve far greater hazard for any aspect of their function. We will look at this more closely.

At the physical level of the energies operating in a human body it is well known that injury and disease can be provoked by other physically stressed agents such as micro-organisms, over exertion and an inappropriate diet, to name but a few of the possibilities. The growth of understanding about such hazards has enabled us to take greater care about them and reduce their effects on health. One particular example is the increased awareness of the sensitivity some children show to certain washing powders or food colourings. Problems with eczema have often been reduced by parents keeping sensitive children away from such provocation.

At the psychological level individual irritants may be less obvious but can be similarly upsetting, particularly if they are unrecognized. As Hahnemann pointed out in the

Organon, words, images and emotions can prove as provocative to susceptible individuals as physically identified stimuli. An example of this provocation occurred in a young woman with a severe anxiety state. Through investigating her anxiety with the help of a psychotherapist she found that it could be precipitated by seeing windows of a certain design. On closer examination she recalled a traumatic interview as a teenager with her school headmistress. The fear felt on that occasion became linked in her memory with the window design. At the time she was too disturbed by the encounter adequately to clarify what was happening to her. She therefore retained a strong but unclear impression of fear associated with the image of the window through which she stared. As a result, in later years, until she traced and clarified the memory imprint, the sight of similar window frames evoked an associated surge of anxiety.

We are all vulnerable to such memories. Non-awareness of them can make us avoid certain situations without understanding why, or leave us vulnerable to their effects if they are aroused. Obviously a greater understanding of such conditioning places us in a far better position to resolve it.

Such examples are far from being the only hazards incurred by a deficiency of self-understanding. Another effect is an inner frustration related to not using our own potential to the full. This may not be so readily apparent as the heightened vulnerability previously described, but again is implied in Hahnemann's writings.[2]

As we noted earlier, health implies wholeness and a full use of our individual functions. This refers not only to obvious physical capabilities, but also to more subtle functions and their role in the development of otherwise hidden capacities. Many times Hahnemann's writings refer to his concern for an efficient pursuit of higher faculties in an on-going evolution. Because of the natural sentience of our organisms there is an innate awareness of their unique functional possibilities. As we noted in the previous chapter, every structure has its own unique intention, form and function. Although they may be masked or repressed during its individual development, they cannot be annihilated. For instance, even people brought up to believe that they cannot paint or draw may sense that skill in themselves, overcome the negative conditioning, and develop such creative arts. Our inborn sensitivity gives a basic awareness of our function in respect to each modality of consciousness. Fulfilment requires its expression;[3] curtailment through non-understanding will incur frustration.

At the level of consciousness usually easiest to observe, that is physical expression, we generally find particular skills emerging in childhood and teenage years. Even with the so-called "late developers", with hindsight early signs are recalled of individual abilities. Obvious examples are athletic and other sporting skills, dexterity with musical instruments, craft or construction work; the list is vast. But whatever their form, the gradual development of such abilities increases personal fulfilment and at the same time demonstrates the interfunction to be realized between all aspects of individual consciousness. Top sportsmen sometimes openly acknowledge that they use psychological training techniques to improve their concentration and physical performance. It is another illustration of the continual interfunction of these aspects of our personality.

When we consider function with an emphasis on sensitivity and reason, again we can often observe signs of their presence in particular individuals from an early age. These too are aspects of our unique form-function whose recognition and employment will give increased personal fulfilment. It may be a natural ability to interpret sound accurately, described as perfect pitch, or an emphasis on attention to detail and a search for explanations, a so-called questioning mind. Other individuals show early signs of a natural ability with languages. These are just a few of the examples of skills placing an emphasis on an individual capacity for accurate, sensitive assessments and similarly precise, reasoned analysis. Here again individuals who possess such abilities find increased personal fulfilment through their expression.

Whatever skills our individual form-function may emphasize, it is, as Hahnemann points out, our own business increasingly to understand and develop them. To restrain them can only incur frustration, like that of a too tightly reined horse. Whereas the contrasting growth of understanding and employment of our potential, brings fulfilment.

But even this level of development, as Hahnemann again reminds us, is not the limit of individual possibilities. Recognizing and exercising a particular ability is one step, the next is further to understand the processes involved both in the performance of the skill and the means by which we can be aware of it. That is, gaining more insight, not only concerning the skill performed, but also of our own ability to reflect and understand how we express it. Used in this way any ability serves as a mirror to help us become more alert to processes operating in our own person. In philosophical terms it has been described as becoming conscious of our consciousness, and it is arguably implicit in Hahnemann's references to self-knowledge.[4] Like many other thinkers Hahnemann argued that through adequate reflection on our personal health, processes operating in disease and the therapies employed to correct them, we can become more aware of our inner consciousness that has developed this outward expression. In previous chapters we have noted many times his recurrent references to the outward activity as being precisely what the term *ex*-pression implies. And similarly, that the consciousness of the inner Self positing this expression is heightened through careful and precise observation of these experiences.

At first such reflection may appear to encourage a selfishness we are often taught to avoid. But if we pursue it thoroughly we see that, far from encouraging a restricting selfish preoccupation, such awareness leads to more understanding of and co-operation with other people. Insight concerning our individual dynamics is the key to more intelligent and effective interaction with other people and our environment. The more we know about ourselves, the more we recognize our interaction with the many aspects of our situation. Self-knowledge therefore becomes a key to giving a more informed and useful response to environmental stimuli. We might refer here to the old maxim that "charity begins at home". It is only through adequate care for our own needs and Self-understanding that we become better placed to help with the needs of others.

Such awareness of individual function and its continuous reciprocal interaction with all other forms of activity, is implicit throughout Hahnemann's writings and arguably reaches a climax in his references to conceptual essences. We noted previously the capacity of a form-function complex to order itself. That is, that the will is integral to the form-function complex expressing it. If we pursue the implications of such an idea in relation to our own being, it implies a similar capacity for self-direction within us. And, further, that such directives can be given in co-operation with the processes of our environment.

This is a profoundly searching concept. On one hand it appears onerous. On the other it endorses individual authority. It removes the self-excuse associated with blaming effects of our own choices on other authorities, but at the same time affirms an essential individual mastery. A growth of such awareness increasingly affirms our capacity to order our own being and to give a progressively appropriate response to the environment in which we live. An early sign of such self-direction occurs when we gain physical control sufficient for walking. More subtle training may be involved later in life if we decide to gain control of personal reactions such as anxiety about driving. Another form of self-direction will be shown if we organize ourselves to study and pursue academic qualifications. All such commitments can be used to pursue Hahnemann's ideal of understanding the processes operating within our own person. If we will, we can use such skills, not only to extend our scope for activity, but also to understand more about our own processes in so doing. Such understanding then places us in a better position to direct our responses to environmental stimuli, and to continue useful activity. It can be a healthy spiral, developing through detailed reflection on our personal processes, and embodying the advice often given by Hahnemann.

The opposite effect is commonly an important factor in the development of disease. If our organism fails to respond adequately or suitably to environmental changes we are vulnerable to unobserved problems. It may be that we fail to see an obstruction and walk into it, or that we fail to understand how a relationship is provoking conflict within us. Ideas, or particular trigger words, may provoke strong reactions if they conflict with our personally preferred data, especially if we are unaware of the processes involved. In all such situations a lack of perception increases our vulnerability, an effect sharply contrasting with the improved health associated with a growing recognition of our essential inner authority.

The development of such authority, it may be argued, is a progressive realization of the unique form-function-volition aspects, or the conceptual essence, of our own being. It implies a growing consciousness of the ways in which our individual dynamic complex can operate here-now. In colloquial terms it is moving towards being able to do "our own thing", where "own" implies true awareness and responsibility for the inner motivation.

A mythological symbol that may be applied here is the double-headed eagle. It reminds us to look in two directions simultaneously. One aspect is the unseen initiative and other psychological determinants of behaviour implied in Hahnemann's references to conceptual essences and the vital forces. The other aspect is the physical organism that incorporates such subtle directives whilst also interacting with factors as gross as diets and drains. All these polar aspects, Hahnemann argues, need continual attention in a pursuit of health. In other words, it is a constant two-way appraisal like that of the double-headed eagle.

The essential aspects of volition-form-function operate within us now, but most of the time we probably realize very little of their true character. Evolution is our gradual re-awakening.

Throughout his work, and his writings describing it, Hahnemann progressively pursued this therapeutic ideal. In the first paragraph of the *Organon* he wrote, "The physician's highest calling, his *only* calling, is to make sick people healthy — to heal, as it is termed."[5] In the following pages, and in many other works, he argued the implications of this ideal in relation to its physical, psychological and volitional or spiritual aspects and the need for their progressive recognition.

Clearly this is an ongoing task. But if we will, we can use our individual state of health or disease to learn more of the processes involved in it. That way we become our own physicians and pursue with Hahnemann and other thinkers the ideal "Know thyself".

REFERENCES

1. *Organon* 6th Edition Para. 141a trans. Künzli, Naudé and Pendleton
2. *Organon* 6th Edition Paras 77, 81a
3. Ibid. Para. 9
4. Ibid. Para. 141 and footnotes
5. *Organon* 6th Edition Para. 1 trans. Künzli, Naudé and Pendleton

INDEX

Index

Tranquillizers, 33
Trituration, 78, 80

Unreasoned reaction of vital
force, 58
Untunement of vital force, 25

Vital force, changes in diseases,
24, 39–40, 41, 43, 58, 62, 64,
67, 107

implications of term, 19, 25,
107
role in maintaining health, 25
role in restoring health, 58–61,
64, 68, 73, 74, 99, 108
Volitional essences, 36, 107, 116,
117

Whooping cough, 43

X-rays, 54